You are only as strong as your core. As a personal trainer, I make core training a foundation for all my clients. You can't get stronger or faster or better at anything without a strong core—and the plank is my go-to move because it's so challenging and versatile. Jen's book should be in every personal trainer's library!

—Leslie Ann Quillen, NASM-CPT; national trainer, Les Mills BODYPUMP®, BODYCOMBAT®

This book is GREAT and perfect for yoga students. Plank pose is a fantastic fitness tool, and this book gives a huge variety of planks that improve posture and give muscles a stabilizing force to add fluidity to yoga practice. It strengthens wrists, neck, and spine, and tones the abs, which give support to the lower back—kind of a perfect pose. This is definitely a book everyone will benefit from.

—Johnna Smith, ParaYoga certified teacher, Baptiste certified teacher, and Certified Ayurvedic Wellness Educator

Ultimate Plank Fitness is jam packed with amazing ways to help you flatten your middle in an entirely new way. Jen not only shows you detailed steps, she walks you through with pictures, making each move easy to follow. This book is a must have for your fitness book collection.

—Heather Connell, R.H.N.C, author of *Powerful Paleo Superfoods* and *Paleo Sweets & Treats*

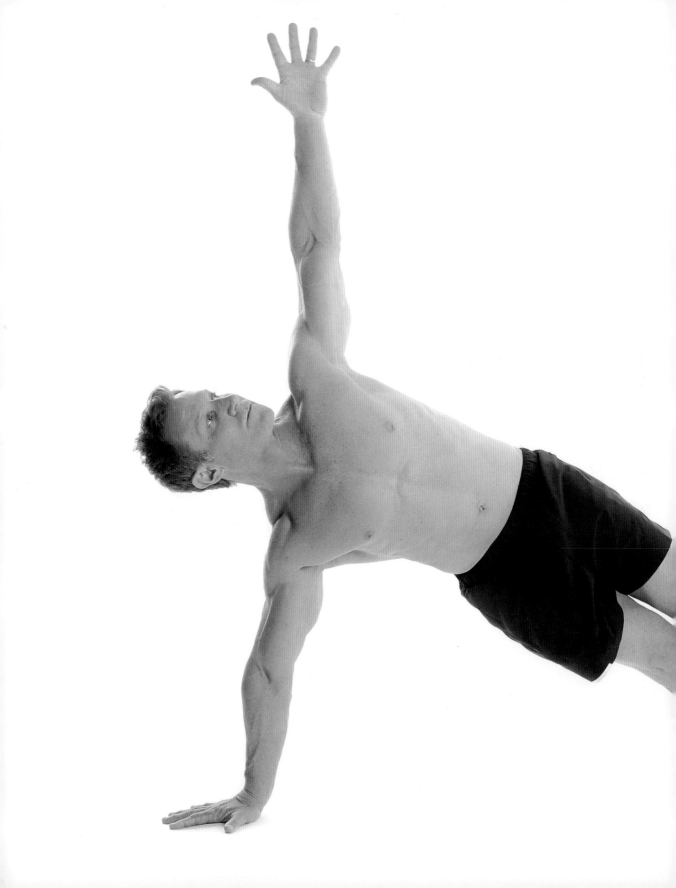

ULTIMATE
PLANK
FITNESS

FOR A STRONG CORE, KILLER ABS—AND A KILLER BODY

JENNIFER DECURTINS

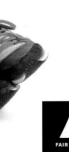

Fair Winds Press
100 Cummings Center, Suite 406L
Beverly, MA 01915

fairwindspress.com • bodymindbeautyhealth.com

© 2015 Fair Winds Press

First published in the USA in 2015 by
Fair Winds Press, a member of
Quarto Publishing Group USA Inc.
100 Cummings Center
Suite 406-L
Beverly, MA 01915-6101
www.fairwindspress.com

Visit www.bodymindbeautyhealth.com.
It's your personal guide to a happy, healthy, and extraordinary life!

18 17 16 15   2 3 4 5

ISBN: 978-1-59233-660-9

Digital edition published in 2015
eISBN: 978-1-62788-305-4

Library of Congress Cataloging-in-Publication Data
DeCurtins, Jen.
        Ultimate plank fitness : for a strong core, killer abs - and a killer body / Jen DeCurtins.
        pages cm
        ISBN 978-1-59233-660-9 (paperback)
        1. Exercise. 2. Physical fitness. 3. Abdominal exercises.
        4. Abdomen--Muscles. 5. Muscle strength. I. Title.

    GV508.D43 2015
    613.7'1--dc23

2014025753

Cover and book design by Mattie S. Wells
Photography by Wanda Koch Photography, www.wandakoch.com
Printed and bound in China

The information in this book is for educational purposes only. It is not intended to replace the advice of a physician or medical practitioner. Please see your health care provider before beginning any new health program.

For my Mema, for opening my eyes
to a world of possibility.

ULTIMATE PLANK FITNESS

PLANK EXERCISE IS A SAFE, CHALLENGING, AND EFFECTIVE METHOD OF CORE CONDITIONING. VARIATIONS OF PLANKS ARE USED ACROSS MANY FITNESS DISCIPLINES, INCLUDING BOOT CAMP REGIMENS, YOGA, PILATES, BARRE, CROSSFIT, AND MANY MORE. THE BENEFITS OF PLANK EXERCISE ARE NUMEROUS. THEY NOT ONLY STRENGTHEN THE ABS BUT ALSO THE ENTIRE CORE AND MANY OTHER MUSCLE GROUPS IN THE UPPER AND LOWER BODY.

WHAT IS THE CORE?

When many people think of core training, the first thing that often comes to mind is sculpting the "six pack," so they focus primarily on training the rectus abdominis (the abs you see when you look in the mirror). In reality, your core is composed of many muscles in the abdomen, hips, back, butt, and legs, and it's necessary to work all of these muscle groups to build a strong core.

THE CORE MUSCLES

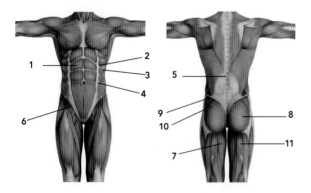

RECTUS ABDOMINIS (1): This is the long, flat muscle that runs the length of the front of the abdomen. The rectus abdominis assists with posture and is responsible for flexing the lumbar spine.

EXTERNAL OBLIQUE (2): This muscle is located along the sides and front of the abdomen and is the largest of the three flat abdominal muscles. The external oblique pulls the chest down to compress the abdominal area and is also important in rotating the trunk.

INTERNAL OBLIQUE (3): This muscle is located along the sides and front of the abdomen, below the external oblique and above the transverse abdominis. When this muscle is contracted, it is responsible for side bending and brings the rib cage closer to the hip. It also aids with trunk rotation.

TRANSVERSE ABDOMINIS (4): Located along the sides and front of the abdominal wall, beneath the internal oblique, this is the deepest layer of the abdominal muscles. It stabilizes the pelvis and the spine, but does not provide any movement.

ERECTOR SPINAE (5): This is a group of three muscles: the iliocostalis, longissimus, and spinalis. They run parallel to each other down the length of the vertebrae, from the sacrum to the neck. The function of the erector spinae is to extend the back (e.g., standing up from a bent-over position) and assist with side-to-side rotation.

HIP FLEXORS (6): This group of muscles is located along the front side of the body, from the abdomen through the top of the thigh. They include the psoas major, iliacus, rectus femoris, pectineus, and sartorius. The hip flexors are responsible for bringing the legs into flexion and in toward the trunk.

HIP ADDUCTORS (7): This group of muscles is located along the inner thigh and includes the adductor brevis, adductor longus, and adductor magnus. They are used in the adduction of the hips (e.g., crossing your legs) and to balance the pelvis while standing and walking.

GLUTEUS MAXIMUS (8): This muscle is located in the buttocks and is the strongest muscle in the human body. It is responsible for movement of the thigh and hip, and many everyday movements, including standing up, maintaining erect posture, and climbing stairs.

GLUTEUS MEDIUS AND GLUTEUS MINIMUS (9): These muscles are located along the side of the hip and buttocks. They facilitate hip abduction and help stabilize the pelvis.

PIRIFORMIS (10): This muscle is located parallel to the gluteus medius and under the gluteus maximus. The function of the piriformis is to laterally rotate the hip.

HAMSTRINGS (11): This muscle group is located along the back of the thigh, starting at the bottom of the pelvis and ending at the lower leg below the knee joint. The group is composed of three muscles: semitendinosus, semimembranosus, and biceps femoris. The hamstrings are responsible for bending and extending at the knee. This muscle group plays an important part in activities such as running, jumping, walking, and more.

BENEFITS OF A STRONG CORE

Think of your core as the trunk of a tree. A strong trunk is the main support system for all of the limbs and branches. When movement of the human body is initiated at the core and then travels to the extremities, this allows your biggest, strongest, and most stable muscles to do the bulk of the work.

BETTER POSTURE: A strong core is essential for good posture, and good posture has a multitude of benefits, ranging from improved breathing quality to better spinal health to projected confidence.

IMPROVED BALANCE AND STABILITY: Balance and stability are an important part of daily life and become even more of a focus as we age. A strong core promotes good balance and a stable, supported body.

STRONGER ATHLETIC PERFORMANCE: Whether you're a runner or a football player, a strong core will enhance your body's athletic ability, resulting in more strength, speed, and stability.

IMPROVED ABILITY TO PERFORM DAILY ACTIVITIES: One of the most basic benefits of a strong core is feeling good in your day-to-day activities, such as running errands, doing yard work, playing with kids, and so on.

ENHANCED JOB PERFORMANCE: There is less discomfort associated with job-related activities when the core is strong, whether that is manual labor or sitting long hours at a desk.

LESS LOWER BACK PAIN: With a strong core, there is less stress and strain placed on the lower back. Think of it like giving yourself a stability belt around the center of the body that keeps all of the muscles and bones in place and functioning correctly.

BENEFITS OF PLANK EXERCISES

STRENGTHEN THE CORE AND WORK UPPER AND LOWER BODY MUSCLES

When you perform plank exercises, you work all of the muscles that make up your core and gain all of the benefits that come with building a strong core. As if that wasn't enough, planks also work the following muscles:

UPPER BODY
- Trapezius
- Rhomboid major and minor
- Rotator cuff
- Anterior, medial, and posterior delts
- Pectorals
- Triceps
- Biceps

LOWER BODY
- Quadriceps
- Gastrocnemius (calf muscle)

PREVENT MUSCLE IMBALANCES

It's easy to develop muscle imbalances when only performing abdominal exercises (such as sit-ups). Most people do not perform spinal and gluteal strengthening exercises to compensate for the abdominal work. Planks condition the front and back of the body simultaneously. When muscles are comparably developed on both sides of the body, the result is better posture, more spinal support, and less lower-back pain.

IMPROVE FUNCTIONAL MOVEMENT

One of the best selling points for planks is their relevance when it comes to functional movement, which is essential movement to living life. Things such as squatting, bending, running, lifting, jumping, and throwing are all functional movements initiated in the core.

PROVIDE A SAFE AND EFFECTIVE ALTERNATIVE TO CRUNCHES AND SIT-UPS

While sit-ups are an important functional movement for daily life (for example, the ability to get out of bed every morning), they are not always the best core conditioning choice for everyone.

Crunches and sit-ups only work the muscles on the front side of the core, so it's necessary to do back strengthening exercises as well. However, planks work the entire core, as well as many other muscles in the body.

Crunches and sit-ups can place pressure on the spine through the repetitive flexion and extension of the spine, and over time, this can become an issue. If you experience any discomfort with these movements, plank training can be a useful substitute.

Furthermore, crunches and sit-ups are counterintuitive for those with ruptured, bulging, or slipped discs or other spinal injuries. Planks are a much safer alternative in these cases.

And finally, crunches and sit-ups can have negative effects on posture by promoting rounded shoulders. Plank exercises promote good posture.

OFFER VERSATILE EXERCISE

The best thing about planks is that there are countless variations of the exercise, ranging from traditional and side plank variations to planks using external weights or unstable surfaces. There is a plank for every body and every fitness level. If one doesn't work for you because of injury, body type, imbalance, or a lack of requisite strength, there are many other options. Entire workouts can be programmed around the plank.

This book features a collection of 101 different variations of planks. The planks are organized by variations, increasing with difficulty and the addition of external props, such as stability balls, gliders, and weights. Each exercise includes a photo demonstration, key performance points, and common faults. The plank descriptions do not focus on time duration; instead, the goal is to fully learn how to perform the plank. Later in the book, to tie it all together, the book ends with ten 5-minute workouts that put what you learn into action with timed workouts that will strengthen the entire core and body.

STANDARD TERMS YOU SHOULD KNOW

Here are a few quick definitions of some standard terms that you'll see throughout the book.

FULL PLANK: This is the starting point for many plank variations in this book. Please reference Full Plank (page 15) for complete instructions.

WORKING SIDE: In side plank variations, the working side is the side of the body in which the hand and foot are grounded to provide stabilization and support.

ENGAGE: When instructed to "engage" a certain body part, squeeze the muscle and maintain continuous contraction of the muscle to support the body.

STACK: This is a position where you create a straight line from one body part to another to form a vertical line. For example, shoulders stacked directly over the wrists or hips stacked on top of one another.

PART ONE

CORE
PLANK
MOVES

This section includes the most basic versions of the plank, which serve as the foundation for building core strength. These planks are performed only with your own bodyweight. Mastering bodyweight planks is an important first step before introducing unstable surfaces and external props.

The planks in this section include the full plank, side plank, forearm plank, and side forearm plank, and variations of each. Once you can confidently perform these basic planks with proper form, you will be ready to move on to the unstable variations and to using external props.

The best thing about the planks featured in this section is that they require no special equipment and can be performed anywhere—at the gym, at home, or as a travel workout. There are many variations of these four planks, ranging from intermediate to advanced, so you won't get bored with your core training.

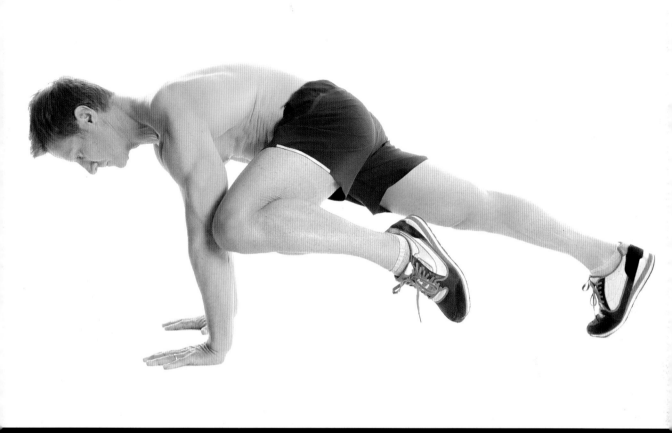

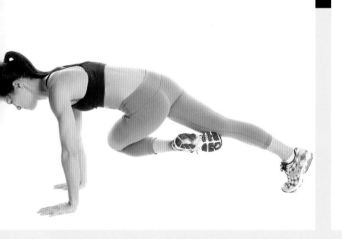

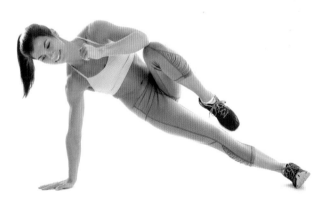

CHAPTER ONE

FULL PLANKS

THE FOUNDATION OF CORE TRAINING

The full plank is the cornerstone of all of the plank variations featured in this book. The ability to hold a stable full plank is a benchmark for fitness and core strength. It's important to practice proper technique as you build the strength necessary to perform a full plank and modifications of it. A strong full plank provides the foundation for moving into progressions involving external weight and unstable surfaces such as stability balls, the BOSU trainer, and medicine balls.

There are many progressions of full plank ranging from beginner to advanced. We will start with the basics and progress through more difficult variations. The planks featured in this chapter are especially appealing because they are simple yet challenging and require no equipment, so they can be performed anywhere.

FULL PLANK

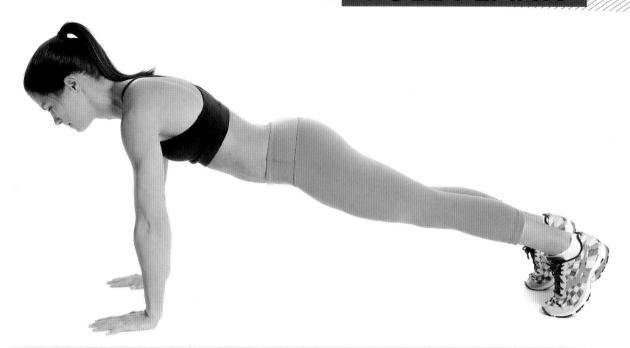

> **SKILL LEVEL: Beginner**

> **MODIFICATION: Can be performed on knees (to make it easier)**

In the full plank, you will maintain a straight body position in a static hold.

KEY PERFORMANCE POINTS

- Start with a straight body position from your head to your heels.
- Stack your shoulders directly over your wrists and firmly plant your palms on the floor.
- Maintain a tight core while squeezing through (also known as "firing through") your quads and your chest to support your core and make the hold easier.

COMMON FAULTS

- Sagging lower back
- Butt lifted higher than the head and heels
- Improper alignment of shoulders and wrists

PAYOFF This is the simplest plank for total core conditioning.

KNEE TO CHEST
FULL PLANK

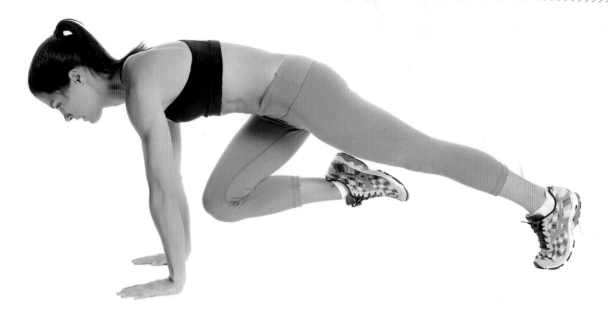

> **SKILL LEVEL: Intermediate**

> **MODIFICATION: Can be performed on knees (to make it easier)**

In the knee-to-chest variation of the full plank, you alternate drawing the knees into the chest.

KEY PERFORMANCE POINTS

- Get into a full plank with a straight body position from your head to your heels with your shoulders stacked over your wrists.
- Lift one foot off the floor and draw your knee into your chest while contracting your abdomen, as if you were performing a crunch. Repeat on the other side for one rep.
- Point your toes and keep your shin parallel to the floor when drawing in your leg.

COMMON FAULTS

- Butt lifted higher than head and heels
- Improper alignment of shoulders and wrists
- Rounding of the upper back

PAYOFF Target and tone the tummy with this knee crunch.

TWISTED KNEE TO CHEST

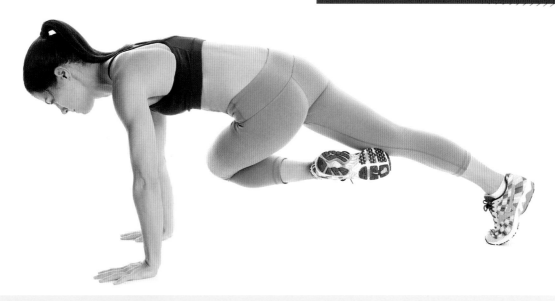

> **SKILL LEVEL: Intermediate**

> **MODIFICATION: Can be performed on knees (to make it easier)**

This variation builds on the knee-to-chest plank by adding in a twist that will tighten and tone the obliques.

KEY PERFORMANCE POINTS

- Estabilish a straight body position from your heels through your head with your gaze down to the floor.

- Stack your shoulders directly over your wrists and plant your palms firmly on the floor.

- Maintain a tight core while firing through your quads and squeezing through your chest to support your core and make the hold easier.

COMMON FAULTS

- Sagging lower back

- Butt lifted higher than your heels and head

- Improper alignment of shoulders and wrists

PAYOFF This plank twists and crunches to tighten abs and obliques.

MOUNTAIN CLIMBER
FULL PLANK

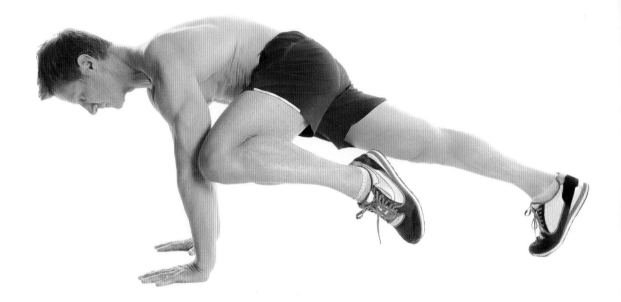

> **SKILL LEVEL: Intermediate**

> **MODIFICATION: Can be performed on knees (to make it easier)**

In the mountain climber variation of full plank, you alternate tapping the knee to the elbow.

KEY PERFORMANCE POINTS

- Get into a full plank with a straight body position from your head to your heels with your shoulders stacked over your wrists.

- Lift one leg off the floor and draw your knee toward your outside elbow and triceps while also contracting your abdomen. Repeat on the other side for one rep.

- Maintain core stability and contract your obliques as your knee draws toward your elbow.

COMMON FAULTS

- Sagging of the body on the non-working side

- Improper alignment of shoulders and wrists

- Rounding of the upper back, shoulders, and wrists

PAYOFF This is a serious oblique sizzler.

SPIDER-MAN

FULL PLANK

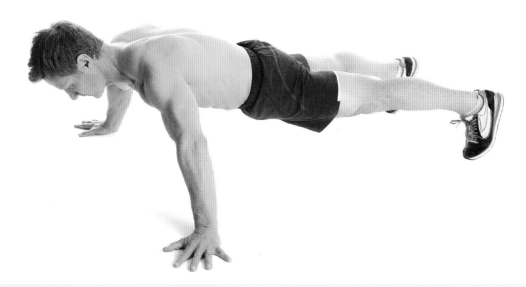

> **SKILL LEVEL: Advanced**

> **MODIFICATION: Can be performed on knees (to make it easier)**

In the Spider-Man variation of full plank, you walk the hands and feet wider than the shoulders and hips while maintaining a static hold. You'll feel this challenging plank variation in the chest, so squeeze those muscles to stay strong.

KEY PERFORMANCE POINTS

- Get into a full plank with a straight body position from your head to your heels with your shoulders stacked over your wrists.

- Place your hands and feet wider than your shoulders and hips. Your elbows should be slightly bent with fingertips facing out.

- Maintain a tight core while squeezing through your quads and your chest to support your core and make the hold easier.

COMMON FAULTS

- Sagging lower back due to the lack of engagement of your chest and core

- Butt lifted higher than head and heels

- Improper hand and foot position

PAYOFF This plank is as effective in working the chest as a push-up.

SPINAL BALANCING

> **SKILL LEVEL: Advanced**

> **MODIFICATION: Can be performed on the knees in a tabletop position (to make it easier)**

The spinal balancing variation of full plank develops control and stabilization in the lumbar region, while the upper and lower body must coordinate to maintain a static hold.

KEY PERFORMANCE POINTS

- Get into a full plank with a straight body position from your head to your heels with your shoulders stacked over your wrists.

- Lift one arm up, and reach it straight out in front of you. Lift the opposite foot. Repeat on the other side for one rep.

- Stack your shoulders directly over your wrists and stabilize through the shoulder that supports the grounded palm.

- Keep your hips square to the floor. Focus on engaging through the lifted arm and leg.

COMMON FAULTS

- Improper alignment of shoulders and wrists

- Hips on the side of the lifted leg higher than your hips on the grounded side

PAYOFF This plank is a serious butt and shoulder burner, and also builds spinal stability.

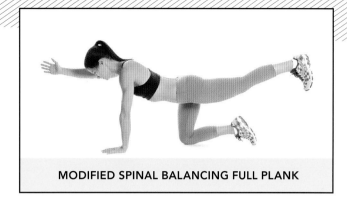

MODIFIED SPINAL BALANCING FULL PLANK

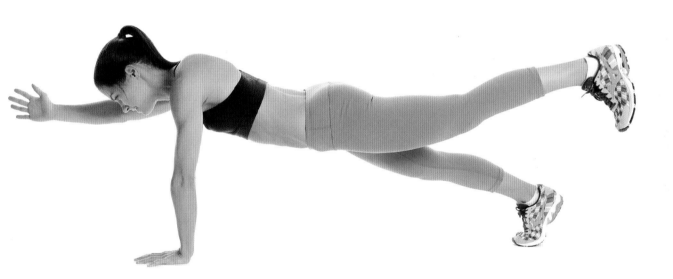

STEPPING

> **SKILL LEVEL: Intermediate**

> **MODIFICATION: Can be performed on knees (to make it easier)**

One way to make a basic plank more difficult is to introduce movement. In this variation, the upper body holds a static plank while the lower body moves with alternating steps in and out with the feet.

KEY PERFORMANCE POINTS

- Get into a full plank with a straight body position from your head to your heels with your shoulders stacked over your wrists.

- Start with your feet apart, about the width of your hips, and then alternate stepping one foot out wider than your hips and back in again. Utilize your hip abductors and adductors to perform the stepping motion. Repeat the process with the other foot for one rep.

- Keep your hips square to the floor as you step your foot out.

COMMON FAULTS

- Sagging lower back

- Butt and hips lifted higher than head and heels, especially on the working side of your body

- Shoulders more forward than your wrists

PAYOFF Movement revs up intensity.

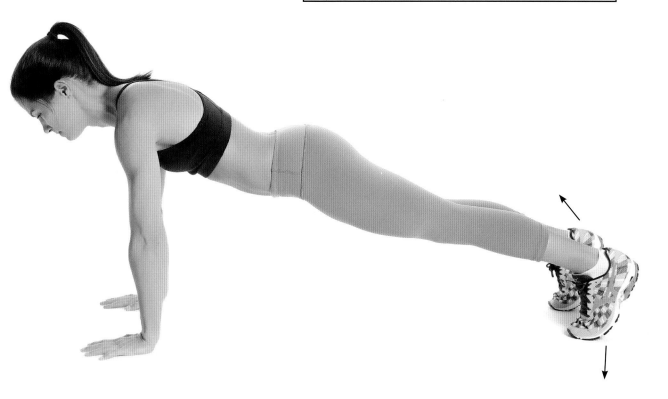

ALTERNATE STEPPING FEET OUT FROM FULL PLANK

PULSING

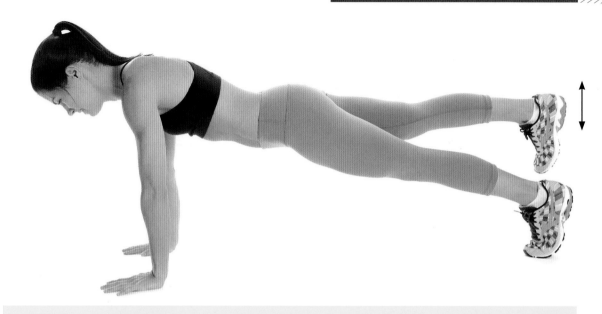

> **SKILL LEVEL: Intermediate**

> **MODIFICATION: Can be performed on knees (to make it easier)**

Get ready to feel the fire in your gluteus with the pulsing plank. This variation of full plank requires the upper body to maintain static position while one leg lifts behind you and performs small pulsing movements.

KEY PERFORMANCE POINTS

- Get into a full plank with a straight body position from your head to your heels with your shoulders stacked over your wrists.
- Lift one foot 6 inches (15 cm) off the floor and perform small pulses up and down. Repeat on the other side for one rep.
- Your feet should be apart—about the width of your hips—and square to the floor throughout the movement.

COMMON FAULTS

- Sagging lower back
- Butt and hips out of alignment with heel and head, especially on the working side
- Shoulders more forward than your wrists

PAYOFF This plank will make you feel the fire in your butt.

ONE ARM

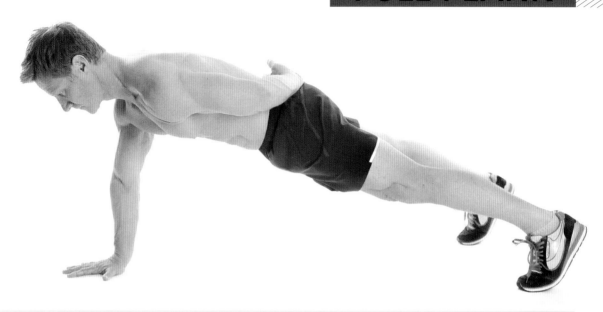

> **SKILL LEVEL: Intermediate**

> **MODIFICATION: Can be performed on knees (to make it easier)**

You remove one point of support in this variation of full plank. One arm will come behind your back as you maintain a static hold.

KEY PERFORMANCE POINTS

- Get into a full plank with a straight body position from your head to your heels with your shoulders stacked over your wrists.

- Shift your weight slightly to one side as you bring one hand behind your back. Press firmly into the palm that is on the floor to stabilize the working shoulder. Repeat on the other side.

- Keep your shoulders and hips square to the floor throughout the movement; placing your feet slightly wider than hip width apart will help you achieve this.

COMMON FAULTS

- Sagging lower back

- Butt and hip out of alignment on non-working side

- Shoulders out of alignment with the wrist

PAYOFF This variation is a major shoulder stabilizer.

WALKS

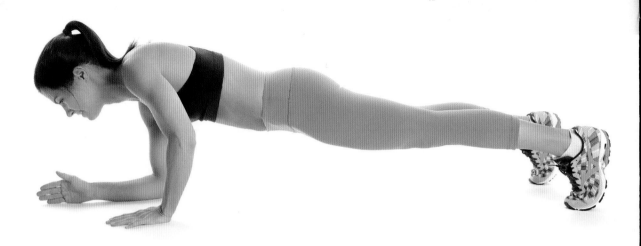

> **SKILL LEVEL: Intermediate**

> **MODIFICATION: Can be performed on knees (to make it easier)**

This variation is a hybrid between a full plank and a forearm plank, where the hands walk from full plank to forearm plank.

KEY PERFORMANCE POINTS

- Get into a full plank with a straight body position from your head to your heels with your shoulders stacked over your wrists.

- Walk your hands from plank to forearm plank and back up to plank again. Repeat on the other side for one rep.

- Keep your hips square to the floor as you perform the walk.

COMMON FAULTS

- Sagging lower back
- Butt lifted higher than head and heels
- Shoulders more forward than your wrists

PAYOFF This exercise turns up the intensity of the full plank.

THREE POINT KNEE TO CHEST

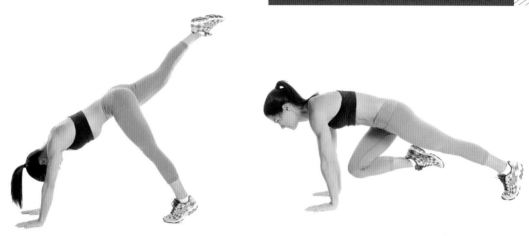

> **SKILL LEVEL:** Intermediate

> **MODIFICATION: Can be performed on knees (to make it easier)**

In this yoga-inspired variation of the full plank, you will move through a range of motions where you extend the working leg high behind you and then draw it in to the chest for what's called a "cheetah crunch."

KEY PERFORMANCE POINTS

- Get into a full plank with a straight body position from your head to your heels with your shoulders stacked over your wrists.

- Push into your palms, and lift your hips to come into an upside down V shape. Lift one leg straight up behind you to come into "three point." Your wrists will be forward of the shoulder when the leg is in three point.

- Point your toes on the lifted leg down and draw the leg into your chest to perform the cheetah crunch.

- Shoulders should stack over your wrists as you draw in for cheetah and reach back to three point.

COMMON FAULTS

- Hip lifted out of alignment on the working side while in three point

- Weight not shifted forward to stack shoulders over wrist while coming in for cheetah crunch

PAYOFF This movement gets your heart rate up and your belly burning.

ARM REACH FRONT AND BACK

FULL PLANK

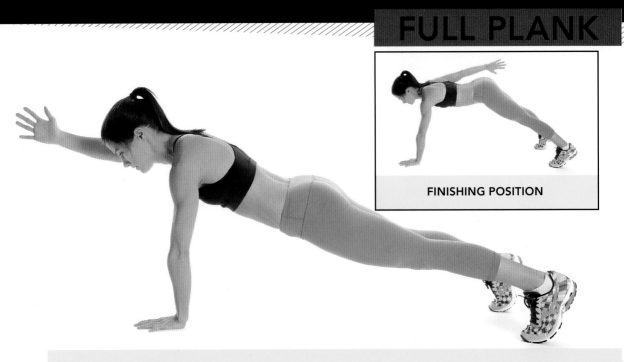

FINISHING POSITION

> **SKILL LEVEL: Intermediate**

> **MODIFICATION: Can be performed on knees (to make it easier)**
>
> This plank requires you to maintain midline stability as you move one arm through a full range of motion by reaching your arm in front of and behind you.

KEY PERFORMANCE POINTS

- Get into a full plank with your shoulders stacked directly over your wrists and slightly wider than your hips.
- Reach one arm straight out in front of you and, as you reach the arm back behind you, lift your hips to create an upside down V-shape with your body.

COMMON FAULTS

- Hip lifted out of alignment on the working side
- Feet in too close
- Improper shoulder alignment

PAYOFF This variation creates killer midline core stability.

DONKEY KICKS

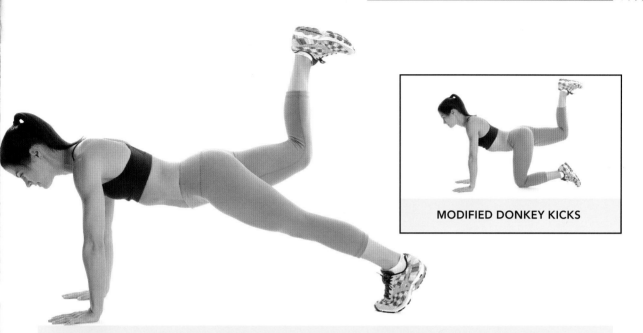

MODIFIED DONKEY KICKS

> **SKILL LEVEL: Intermediate**

> **MODIFICATIONS: Can be performed on knees (to make it easier), or add some tiny pulses (to make it harder)**

In this variation, adding the donkey kick to a static plank hold provides an extra challenge for the gluteus and hamstrings.

KEY PERFORMANCE POINTS

- Get into a full plank with your shoulders stacked over your wrists, and gaze down at the floor.
- Lift one leg behind you, bent at the knee with your heel pointed toward the ceiling.
- Lift the heel toward the ceiling by engaging your hamstrings and gluteus; then lower the heel back down so that the knees align. This is one rep.

COMMON FAULTS

- Improper position of the lifted leg
- Butt lifted higher than head and heels
- Shoulders more forward than the wrist

PAYOFF This plank lifts your butt and sculpts your hamstrings.

FULL PLANKS // 29

INCHWORMS

> **SKILL LEVEL:** Intermediate

> **MODIFICATION:** None

This plank introduces a walking motion with the hands that requires core control and stretches the hamstrings. Do it early in your workout to warm up the body.

KEY PERFORMANCE POINTS

- Get into a full plank with a straight body position from your head to your heels with your shoulders stacked over your wrists.

- Walk your hands back toward your feet while keeping your knees as straight as possible. Draw your abs in and up to facilitate this movement.

- Once your hands have reached your feet, walk your hands back out to a high plank position, bracing your abs as you move.

COMMON FAULTS

- Bent knees on the walk up and down, which doesn't stretch the hamstring

- Shoulders more forward than the wrists

PAYOFF This plank offers both stretching and lengthening of the body.

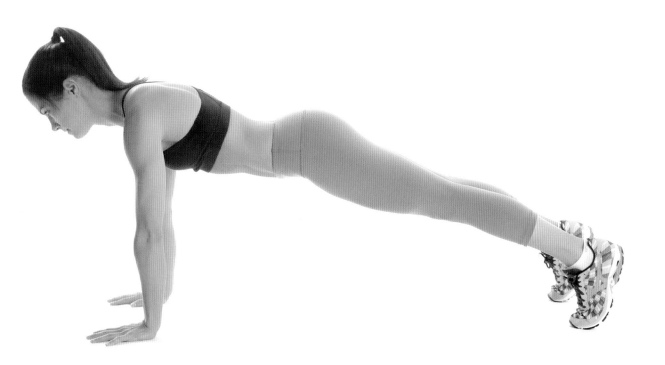

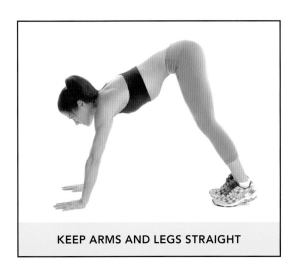

KEEP ARMS AND LEGS STRAIGHT

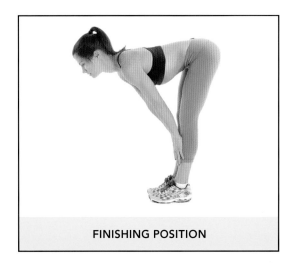

FINISHING POSITION

FULL PLANK

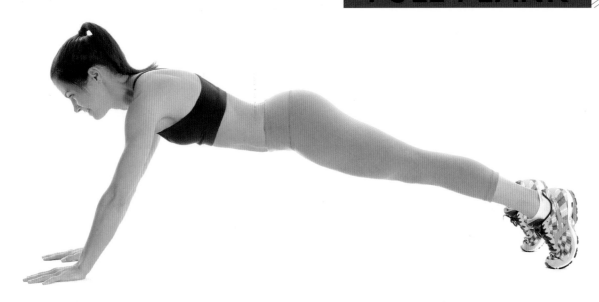

> **SKILL LEVEL: Intermediate**

> **MODIFICATION: Can be performed on knees (to make it easier)**

Adding a walkout with the hands to a static plank creates a whole new challenge for the abdominal wall. Get ready to really brace the core and feel some shaking.

KEY PERFORMANCE POINTS

- Get into a full plank with a straight body position from your head to your heels with your shoulders stacked over your wrists.

- Slowly walk your hands out in front of your head so that your wrists are about a foot in front of your shoulders. Then, walk your hands back to the full plank position.

- Make it easier to maintain square hips and a straight body position throughout the movement by placing your feet slightly wider than your hips.

COMMON FAULTS

- Butt lifted higher than head and heels

- Bent elbows during the walkout

- Sagging lower back

PAYOFF This plank builds a rock-solid abdominal wall.

FULL PLANK

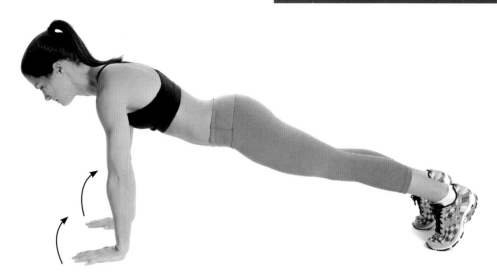

> **SKILL LEVEL: Intermediate**

> **MODIFICATION: Can be performed on knees (to make it easier)**

In this variation of a full plank, the feet remain static while the hands walk around in a semicircle or full circle (depending on space) and then back to the starting position to complete one rep.

KEY PERFORMANCE POINTS

- Get into a full plank with a straight body position from your head to your heels with your shoulders stacked over your wrists.

- Walk your hands in one direction by bringing one arm out to the side and then the other in to meet it, repeating this pattern until you perform a semicircle or full circle (depending on space), and walk back in the opposite direction.

- Make it easier to maintain square hips and a straight body position throughout the movement by taking your feet slightly wider than your hips.

COMMON FAULTS

- Sagging lower back

- Bent elbows during the walking phase

- Butt lifted higher than head and heels

PAYOFF This plank tones the chest and shoulders while also working the abs.

SHOULDER TAP

FULL PLANK

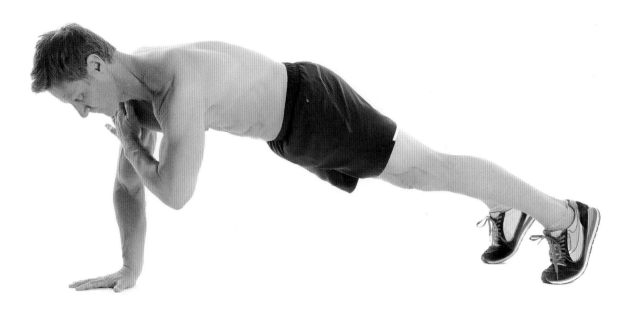

> **SKILL LEVEL: Advanced**

> **MODIFICATION: Can be performed on knees (to make it easier)**

In this variation of a full plank, you alternate lifting one arm and tapping the opposite shoulder. This is an advanced variation that requires a ton of stability and body control.

KEY PERFORMANCE POINTS

- Get into a full plank with a straight body position from your head to your heels with your shoulders stacked over your wrists.

- Lift one hand and tap the opposite shoulder; repeat on the other side.

- Make it easier to maintain square hips and a straight body position throughout the movement by placing your feet slightly wider than your hips.

COMMON FAULTS

- Sagging lower back
- Bent elbows on the grounded arm
- Butt lifted higher than head and heels

PAYOFF This plank builds dynamic body control.

CHAPTER TWO

SIDE PLANKS

DEVELOP SHOULDER STABILIZATION AND SCULPT YOUR WAIST

Now that you've mastered the full plank, the next step is to tackle side plank variations. While you are still working with body weight only, with side planks you are generally working with only one point of support on both the hands and feet.

The benefits of incorporating side planks into your training routine include building strength in the obliques, stabilizing the shoulders, and improving overall core control. Side planks also strengthen the wrists, butt, and thighs.

The variations of side planks in this chapter require no equipment and can be performed anywhere.

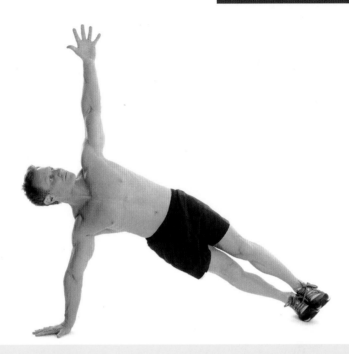

> **SKILL LEVEL: Beginner**

> **MODIFICATIONS: Can be performed on one knee or with split feet (to make it easier)**

This is the most basic side plank, the one that all other side planks in the book will progress from. It requires you to maintain a static hold in a full side plank.

KEY PERFORMANCE POINTS

- Place the working hand on the floor directly underneath the shoulder, and press into the palm to stabilize the shoulder joint.
- Stack your hips and feet on top of one another to create a straight line from your head to your heels.
- Extend the arm of the lifted side straight up and actively drive through your hips to lift the side of your body.

COMMON FAULTS

- Side body sagging
- Hips rotated forward or backward
- Hand placement more forward than the shoulder

PAYOFF This is the most basic way to sculpt your side body.

FOOT TAPS

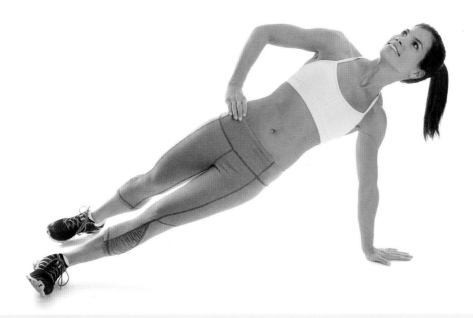

> **SKILL LEVEL: Intermediate**

> **MODIFICATION: Can be performed on one knee (to make it easier)**

In this variation, subtle movement is added to the static side plank hold to challenge shoulder and abdominal stabilization.

KEY PERFORMANCE POINTS

- Place the working hand on the floor directly underneath the shoulder, and press into the palm to lift through the side body.

- Stack your hips and feet on top of one another to create a straight line from your head to your heels. Place the non-working hand on the top hip.

- Lift your top leg up a few inches. Then alternate tapping your foot in front of and behind the grounded leg while maintaining a strong core and stabilized shoulder.

COMMON FAULTS

- Side body sagging

- Bent knee on working leg

- Hand placement more forward than the shoulder

PAYOFF This variation trains the shoulder stabilization throughout the movement.

WITH HIP DIPS

> **SKILL LEVEL: Intermediate**

> **MODIFICATION: Feet can be split (to make it easier)**

Movement is introduced in the side plank by dipping the hips down and up for a great variation that makes you feel the burn in your obliques.

KEY PERFORMANCE POINTS

- Place the working hand on the floor directly underneath the shoulder, and press into the palm to lift through the side body.
- Stack your hips and feet on top of one another to create a straight line from your head to your heels.
- Dip your hips and lifted arm down toward the floor, then engage through the top side of your body to lift them back up as high as you can while you reach your arm up.

COMMON FAULTS

- Hips and shoulders rotated forward or backward
- Hand placement more forward than the shoulder

PAYOFF This plank creates definition in the obliques.

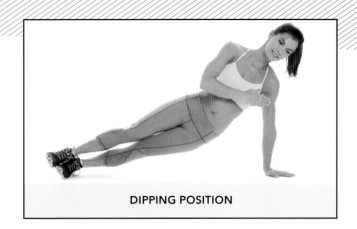

DIPPING POSITION

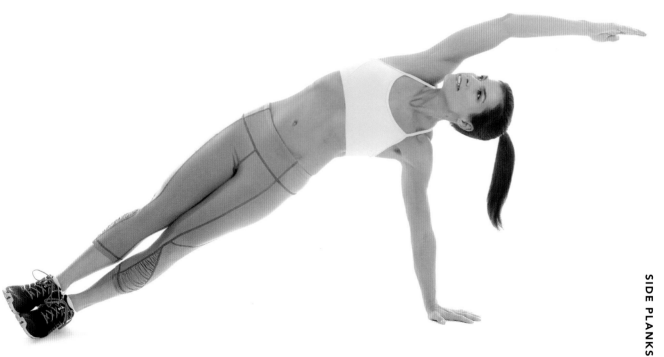

TREE

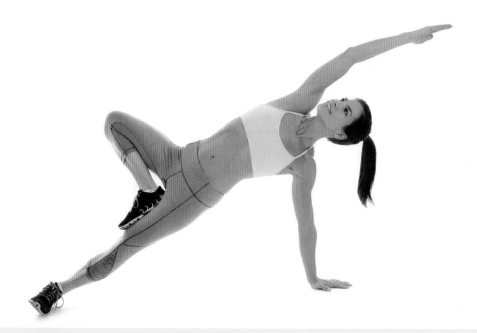

> **SKILL LEVEL:** Intermediate

> **MODIFICATION:** Can be performed on one knee (to make it easier)

Add the yoga pose tree to the side plank to test your balance and stability as you perform a static hold.

KEY PERFORMANCE POINTS

- Place the working hand on the floor directly underneath the shoulder, and press into the palm to lift through the side body.
- Stack your hips and feet on top of one another to create a straight line from your head to your heels.
- Bend your top leg, and place your foot either to the inside of the shin or thigh, pointing your knee toward the ceiling. Reach the non-working arm over your head with your bicep over your ear.

COMMON FAULTS

- Foot placed on knee joint
- Hips rotated forward or backward
- Hand placement more forward than the shoulder

PAYOFF This plank challenges balance and stability while gently stretching the side body.

LEG RAISE

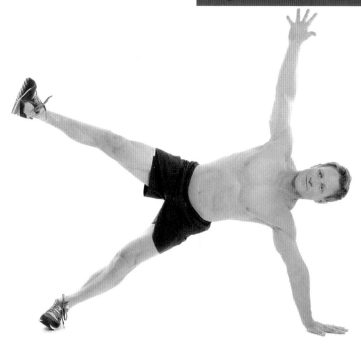

> **SKILL LEVEL: Intermediate**

> **MODIFICATION: Can be performed on one knee (to make it easier)**

Add a leg lift to your plank to boost the challenge for your obliques and add some work for your hips.

KEY PERFORMANCE POINTS

- Place the working hand on the floor directly underneath the shoulder, and press into the palm to lift through the side body.

- Stack your hips and feet on top of one another to create a straight line from your head to your heels.

- Lift your top leg up as high as you can while engaging the lifted leg, abs, and working shoulder. Reach the non-working arm straight up toward the ceiling.

COMMON FAULTS

- Side body sagging

- Hips rotated forward or backward

- Hand placement more forward than the shoulder

PAYOFF This plank whittles away at the waistline.

STAR

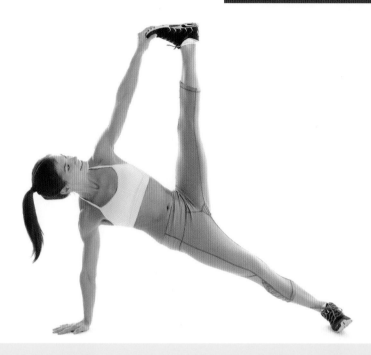

> **SKILL LEVEL: Advanced**

> **MODIFICATION: Can be performed on one knee (to make it easier); the lifted knee can be bent (if flexibility isn't there)**

This advanced variation of side plank requires both strong midline stability and flexibility as you maintain a static hold.

KEY PERFORMANCE POINTS

- Place the working hand on the floor directly underneath the shoulder, and press into the palm to lift through the side body.
- Stack your hips and feet on top of one another to create a straight line from your head to your heels.
- Bend your knee and grasp the toe area of the shoe, then reach your heel away to straighten the leg.
- Lift your hips as high as you can while maintaining a static hold; gaze either straight ahead or toward the lifted leg.

COMMON FAULTS

- Side body sagging
- Hips rotated forward
- Hand placement more forward than the shoulder

PAYOFF This is a huge test of flexibility and total body strength.

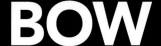
BOW

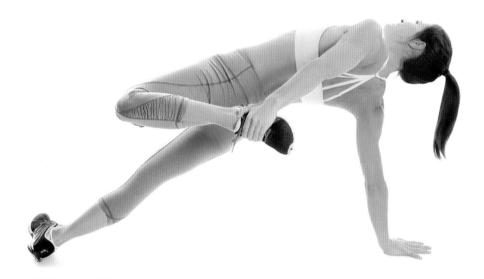

> **SKILL LEVEL: Advanced**

> **MODIFICATION: Can be performed on one knee (to make it easier)**

This is another advanced variation requiring strength and flexibility. This variation requires a backbend while also maintaining a static hold in side plank.

KEY PERFORMANCE POINTS

- Place the working hand on the floor directly underneath the shoulder, and press into the palm to lift through the side body.

- Stack your hips and feet on top of one another to create a straight line from your head to your heels.

- Draw the top knee in toward your chest, and wrap the lifted hand around your ankle.

- Keeping the hand and foot together, press your heel back behind you while also opening your chest and lifting through your hips.

COMMON FAULTS

- Side body sagging
- Shoulder rotated forward
- Hand placement more forward than the shoulder

PAYOFF This variation opens the chest and upper back while also building total body strength.

SIDE PLANK WITH KNEE CRUNCHES

> **SKILL LEVEL:** Intermediate

> **MODIFICATION:** Can be performed on knees (to make it easier)

The addition of a knee crunch provides a two-for-one benefit: working the abs and obliques at the same time.

KEY PERFORMANCE POINTS

- Place the working hand on the floor directly underneath the shoulder, and press into the palm to lift through the side body.
- Stack your hips and feet on top of one another to create a straight line from your head to your heels.
- Lift your top leg up a few inches, and then draw your knee and lifted elbow into your chest. Then, reach both away, fully straightening and extending.

COMMON FAULTS

- Side body sagging
- Hips and shoulders rotated forward or backward
- Hand placement more forward than the shoulder

PAYOFF This plank creates six-pack abs and chiseled obliques.

CRUNCHING POSITION

SIDE PLANK

SIDE PLANK

> **SKILL LEVEL: Intermediate**

> **MODIFICATION: Can be performed on one knee or with split feet (to make it easier)**

This variation of side plank builds not only a strong core, but an upper body as well. You will alternate between performing a push-up and a side plank.

KEY PERFORMANCE POINTS

- Place the working hand on the floor directly underneath the shoulder, and press into the palm to lift through the side body.

- Stack your hips and feet on top of one another to create a straight line from your head to your heels.

- Bring the lifted side down to a full plank and perform a push-up (on your toes, for more difficulty, or on your knees, to make it easier) and then rotate into the side plank on the opposite side.

COMMON FAULTS

- Not maintaining straight body position throughout the plank and push-up

- Hand placement more forward than the shoulder

PAYOFF This variation adds a push-up to tone and strengthen the upper body.

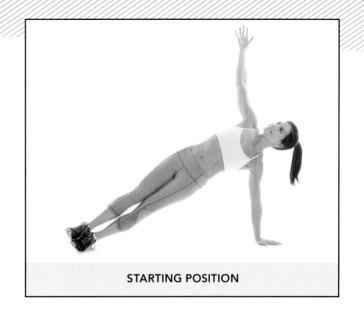

STARTING POSITION

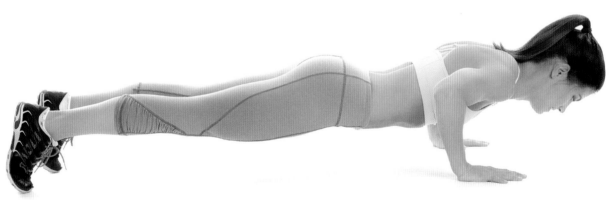

CHAPTER THREE

FOREARM PLANKS

INCREASE YOUR RESISTANCE TO AMP UP INTENSITY

In this chapter, everything comes back to center with forearm planks. This is a progression of your full plank; all of the same mechanics and rules of full plank apply, but here you work from the forearms instead of the hands.

Incorporating forearm planks into your training is beneficial because as your center of gravity moves closer to the floor, your core must work harder to support your bodyweight.

Forearm planks are also ideal variations for individuals with wrist problems or pain. The variations of forearm planks in this chapter use bodyweight only and require no equipment.

FULL

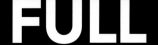

FOREARM PLANK

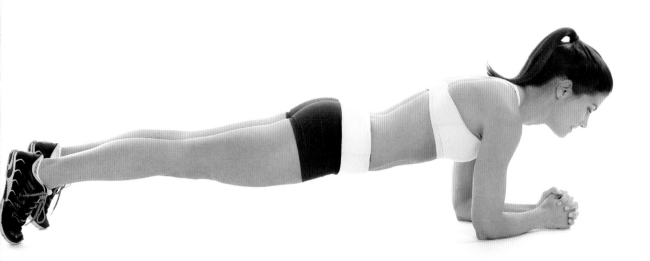

> **SKILL LEVEL: Beginner**
> **MODIFICATION: Can be performed on knees (to make it easier)**
> In the forearm plank, you maintain a straight body position in a static hold.

KEY PERFORMANCE POINTS

- Get into a straight body position from your head through your heels.
- Stack your shoulders directly over your elbows, and press into your forearms to support your shoulders.
- Maintain a tight core while squeezing through your quads and chest.

COMMON FAULTS

- Sagging lower back
- Butt lifted higher than the head and heels
- Improper alignment of shoulders and elbows

PAYOFF In this variation, bring your bodyweight closer to the floor to up the intensity.

ROCKING

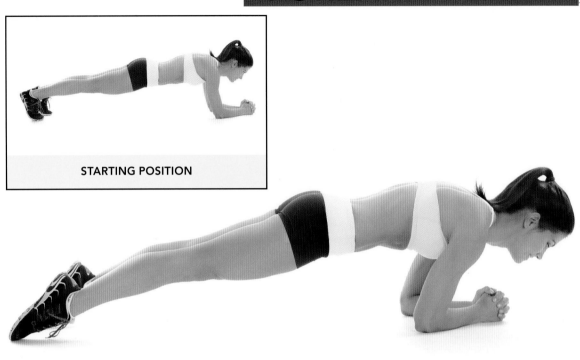

STARTING POSITION

> **SKILL LEVEL: Beginner**

> **MODIFICATION: None**

Slight movement is introduced in this variation for an additional core challenge.

KEY PERFORMANCE POINTS

- Get into a straight body position from your head through your heels with your shoulders stacked over your forearms.
- Press through your toes and back through your heels to perform a rocking motion.

COMMON FAULTS

- Sagging lower back
- Bent knees
- Butt lifted higher than the head and heels

PAYOFF Rock back and forth for rock solid abs.

KNEE TAPS

FOREARM PLANK

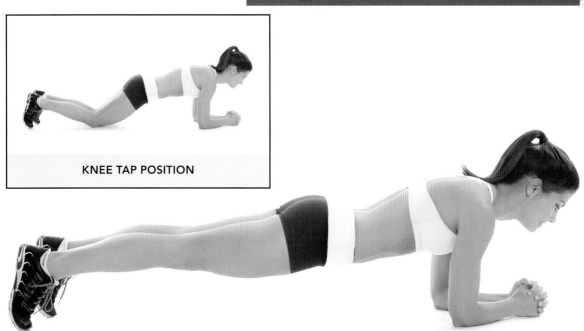

KNEE TAP POSITION

> **SKILL LEVEL: Beginner**

> **MODIFICATION: None**

This is another variation that plays with slight movement to build core stability.

KEY PERFORMANCE POINTS

- Get into a straight body position from your head through your heels with your shoulders stacked over your forearms.
- Tap your knees to the floor, and then squeeze through your quads to straighten your legs.

COMMON FAULTS

- Sagging lower back
- Butt lifted higher than the head and heels
- Shoulders more forward than the forearms

PAYOFF This variation strengthens the core, shoulders, quads, and hamstrings.

HIP DROPS

FOREARM PLANK

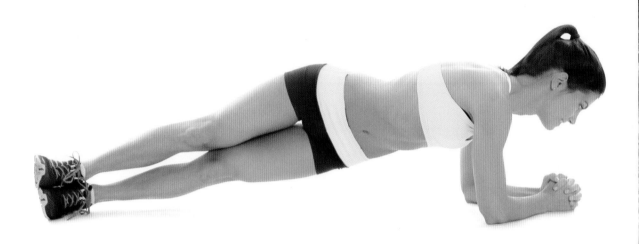

> **SKILL LEVEL: Intermediate**

> **MODIFICATION: None**

In this variation, you'll add a side-to-side hip drop to define the waist. This variation requires maximum core engagement.

KEY PERFORMANCE POINTS

- Get into a straight body position from your head through your heels with your shoulders stacked over your forearms.
- Alternate dipping your hips from side to side. As you do this, roll to the sides of your feet.

COMMON FAULTS

- Sagging lower back
- Butt lifted higher than the head and heels
- Shoulders more forward than the forearms

PAYOFF This plank slims the waist.

CROSSOVER
FOREARM PLANK

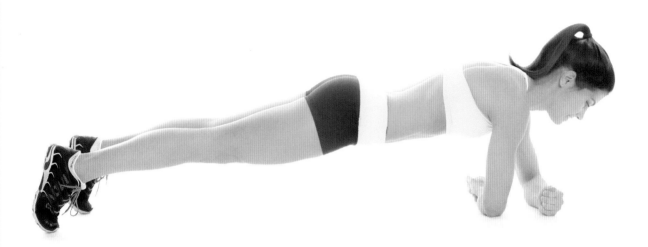

> **SKILL LEVEL: Intermediate**

> **MODIFICATION: Can be performed on knees (to make it easier)**

This forearm plank introduces movement of the arms while you keep the core and lower body stable and static.

KEY PERFORMANCE POINTS

- Get into a straight body position from your head to your heels.
- Stack your shoulders directly over your elbows, and turn your forearms so that they are parallel with one another.
- Walk one forearm in front of the other and back to starting position; repeat on both sides for one rep.

COMMON FAULTS

- Sagging lower back
- Butt lifted higher than the head and heels
- Shoulders more forward than the forearms

PAYOFF This plank gets the shoulders and triceps working.

AROUND THE WORLD MARCHING

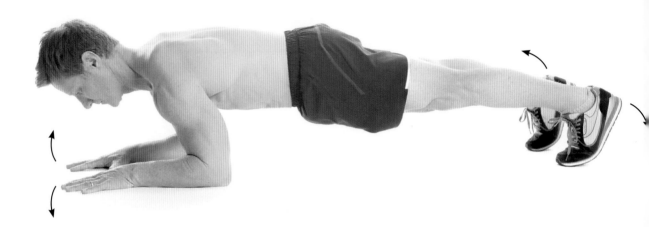

> **SKILL LEVEL: Advanced**

> **MODIFICATION: None**

In this advanced variation of the forearm plank, both the arms and legs are in movement to create a true challenge of core stabilization.

KEY PERFORMANCE POINTS

- Get into a straight body position from your head through your heels with your shoulders stacked over your forearms.
- While maintaining forearm plank position, alternate reaching your right hand out, tapping the floor, and bringing it back to the starting position. Then reach your left hand out and back to the starting position. Then reach your right foot out and back to the starting position, and finally your left foot out and back to the starting position. This is one rep.

COMMON FAULTS

- Sagging lower back
- Butt lifted higher than the head and heels
- Shoulders more forward than the forearms

PAYOFF The double movement of this plank introduces a massive stabilization challenge.

DOLPHIN

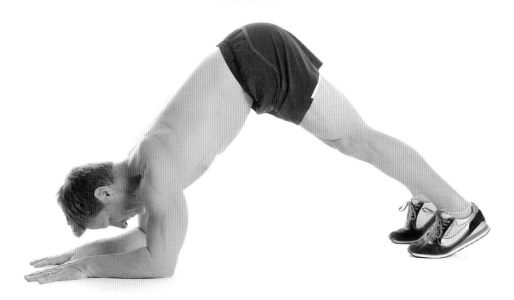

> **SKILL LEVEL: Beginner**

> **MODIFICATION: None**

In the dolphin variation of forearm plank, there is an intentional lifting of the butt higher than the heels and head, where you will then maintain a static hold. This variation develops upper body strength and trains you to draw your abdominal muscles in and up.

KEY PERFORMANCE POINTS

- Get into a straight body position from your head through your heels with your shoulders stacked over your forearms.
- Walk your feet as close up to your knees as possible as you lift through your abs and gluteus.
- Maintain a static hold as you squeeze through your quads to help support your abs, and keep your gaze neutral toward the floor.

COMMON FAULTS

- Holding your breath
- Bent knees

PAYOFF This plank works the lats and upper back while pulling in the abs.

PLANK PUSH-UP

> **SKILL LEVEL: Advanced**

> **MODIFICATION: None**

With this variation, you build on the dolphin plank by adding movement to perform dolphin push-ups. Rock the body front and back for one rep.

KEY PERFORMANCE POINTS

- Place your forearms on the floor directly under your shoulders, and create a straight line from elbow to wrist. Press into your forearms to support your shoulders.

- Walk your feet as close up to your knees as possible as you lift through your abs and gluteus. This is the dolphin plank position.

- Bring your body out to a forearm plank and then lift back up into the dolphin plank. This is one rep.

COMMON FAULTS

- Bent knees

PAYOFF This variation is guaranteed to give you a burn as you tighten and tone both the upper body and abs.

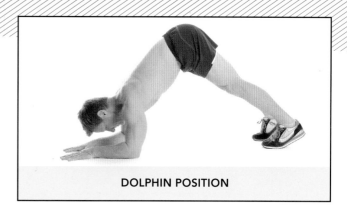

DOLPHIN POSITION

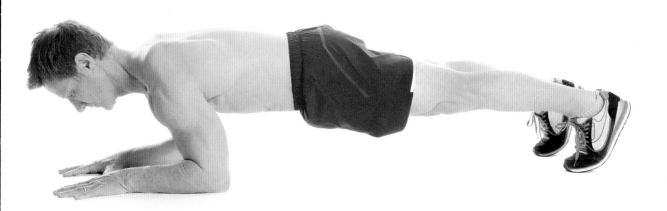

CHAPTER FOUR

SIDE FOREARM PLANKS

SHRED YOUR OBLIQUES

This chapter focuses on side variations of the forearm plank, similar to the full side planks in chapter 2. Even though side forearm planks can feel more challenging than the traditional side plank (because your bodyweight is closer to the floor), they feel more supportive for most people. This is because you have more contact with the floor, since the forearm, instead of just the palm, is pressed into the floor. Side forearm planks are a great option for those who experience wrist pain or weakness with full side plank.

The variations of side forearm plank in this chapter use bodyweight only and require no equipment.

SIDE FOREARM PLANK

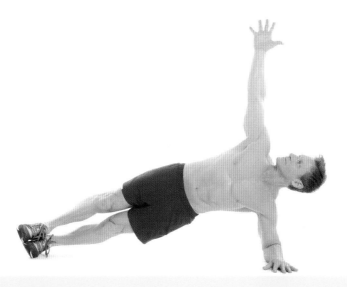

> **SKILL LEVEL: Beginner**

> **MODIFICATION: Can be performed on one knee or with split feet (to make it easier)**

This is the cornerstone side forearm plank from which all other side forearm planks in the book will progress. This exercise requires you to maintain a static hold in a side forearm plank with a stacked body position.

KEY PERFORMANCE POINTS

- Align your shoulder directly over your elbow; press into your forearm to support the shoulder joint.
- Stack your hips and feet on top of one another to create a straight line from your head to your heels, and actively lift the side of your body up as high as possible.
- Extend the arm of the lifted side straight up; actively lift the side body up as high as possible.

COMMON FAULTS

- Side body sagging
- Hips rotated forward or backward
- Elbow placement not in line with shoulder

PAYOFF This plank slims the waist and strengthens the side body.

WRIST GRAB

SIDE FOREARM PLANK

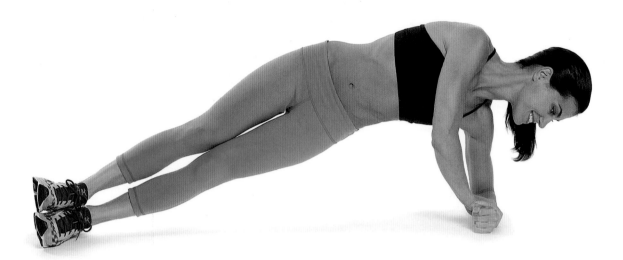

> **SKILL LEVEL: Beginner**

> **MODIFICATION: Can be performed on one knee or with split feet (to make it easier)**

This variation is very similar to the basic side forearm plank, but you will rotate the chest and shoulder down a little bit and close the chest to be sure that you really use the obliques to perform the side forearm plank.

KEY PERFORMANCE POINTS

- Align your shoulder directly over your elbow; press into your forearm to support the shoulder joint.
- Stack your hips and feet on top of one another to create a straight line from your head to your heels, and actively lift the side of your body up as high as possible.
- Reach the hand on the lifted side down to wrap around the grounded wrist. Slightly rotate your chest and shoulders down, and gaze at your fist.

COMMON FAULTS

- Side body sagging
- Hips rotated forward or backward
- Elbow placement not in line with shoulder

PAYOFF This plank slims the waist and strengthens the side body.

HIP DIPS

SIDE FOREARM PLANK

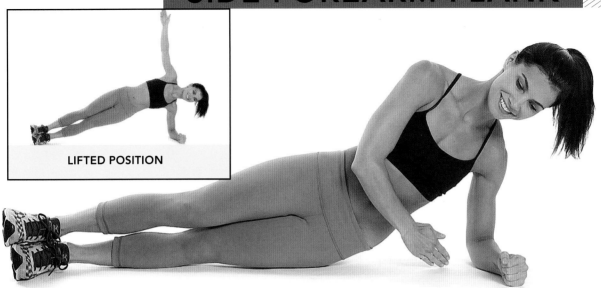

LIFTED POSITION

> **SKILL LEVEL: Intermediate**

> **MODIFICATION: Can be performed with split feet (to make it easier)**

Movement is introduced in this exercise with a hip dipping and lifting motion that will recruit the obliques to work even harder. One dip down and lift up is a rep.

KEY PERFORMANCE POINTS

- Align your shoulder directly over your elbow; press into your forearm to support the shoulder joint.
- Stack your hips and feet on top of one another to create a straight line from your head to your heels, and actively lift the side of your body up as high as possible.
- Dip your hips and lifted hand down toward the floor, and then engage through your hips and obliques. Lift them back up as high as you can while you reach your hand up.

COMMON FAULTS

- Hips rotated forward or backward
- Elbow placement not in line with shoulder

PAYOFF This plank whittles away at the waistline.

ROLLING

> **SKILL LEVEL: Intermediate**

> **MODIFICATION: Can be performed on knees (to make it easier)**

All of the movement here is in the upper body as you rotate elbow and chest down toward the hand and rotate open again while maintaining a strong side forearm plank.

KEY PERFORMANCE POINTS

- Align your shoulder directly over your elbow; press into your forearm to support the shoulder joint.

- Stack your hips and feet on top of one another to create a straight line from your head to your heels, and actively lift the side of your body up as high as possible.

- Bring the hand of the lifted arm behind your head. Slowly roll your elbow down toward the grounded hand. Roll back up to full extension to complete the movement.

COMMON FAULTS

- Sagging hips during the movement

- Hips rotated forward or backward

- Elbow placement not in line with shoulder

PAYOFF The rotation in this exercise recruits more muscles to work.

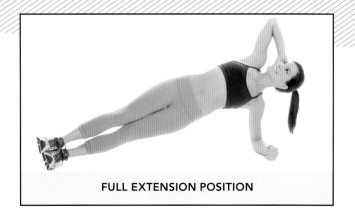

FULL EXTENSION POSITION

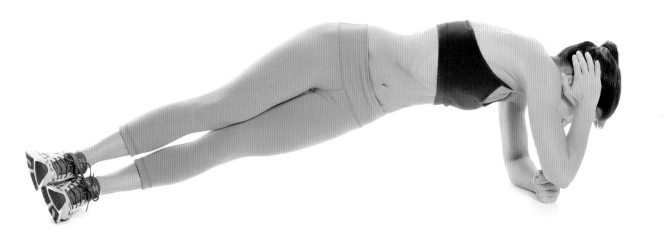

PART TWO

UNSTABLE SURFACE

PLANKS

Now that you've perfected bodyweight planks, it's time to introduce unstable surfaces. The unstable surfaces used in this chapter include stability balls, BOSU Trainers, and medicine balls. These items can commonly be found in gyms and are great equipment to own if you have a home gym.

HERE ARE SOME OF THE MANY BENEFITS TO ADDING UNSTABLE SURFACES TO YOUR CORE TRAINING:

INCREASES YOUR NEUROMUSCULAR EFFICIENCY. Neuromuscular efficiency is the ability of the neuromuscular system to work in union to produce and reduce force and dynamically stabilize the body. Using unstable surfaces is one of the fastest ways to build the communication efficiency between the nervous and muscular systems in the body. Simply put, you're improving your mind-body connection.

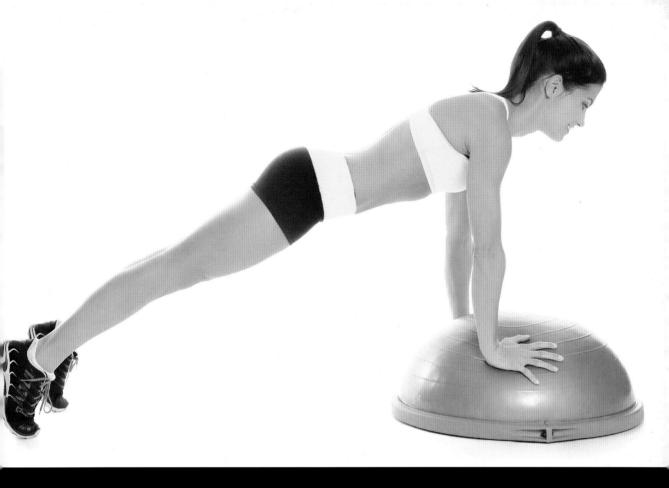

IMPROVES BALANCE AND COORDINATION. Unstable surfaces require the body to be on call and ready for action. When working on an unstable surface, the muscles are constantly working to stabilize and maintain position.

CONDITIONS DEEP STABILIZER MUSCLES. The core includes some deep stabilizing muscles, including the rectus abdominis, transverse abdominis, oblique abdominis, and erector spinae. Unstable surfaces require you to recruit these muscles that can otherwise be difficult to target.

Grab an unstable prop and get ready to take your core stabilization to the next level.

FULL PLANK

CHAPTER FIVE

STABILITY BALL
PLANKS

DEVELOP BALANCE AND COORDINATION

The first unstable surface that you will work with in the unstable surface progression is the stability ball. The stability ball is the big beach ball–like thing you see in gyms. It's also great for home gym use because it's so versatile. Stability balls have become popular due to their multitude of benefits. They work the entire core, including the abdomen, lower back, gluteus, and thighs, and they also increase spinal stability, balance, and coordination.

These plank variations are more challenging than their stable counterparts, so introduce them only after you have a solid full plank. When you sit on the ball, the hips should be level or slightly higher than the knees. Here's a general reference guide for the size of ball you'll need based on your height:

55 cm — 4'11"– 5'4" | 65 cm — 5'5"– 5'11" | 75 cm — 6'0"– 6'7"
   (150–163 cm)   (164–180 cm)   (181–200 cm)

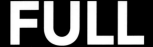
FULL

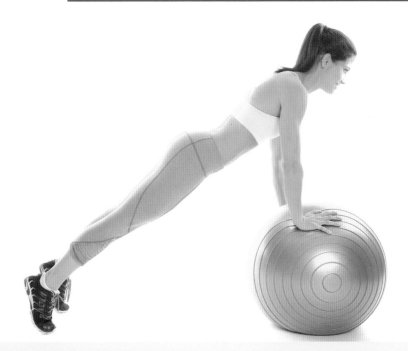

> **SKILL LEVEL: Intermediate**

> **MODIFICATION: Place stability ball against a stable service like a wall (for more support)**

In the stability ball plank, you will maintain a static hold in a full plank position with your hands on the stability ball and feet on the floor.

KEY PERFORMANCE POINTS

- Get into a straight body position from your head to your heels.
- Stack your shoulders over your wrists; firmly plant your palms on either side of the stability ball.
- Maintain a tight core while squeezing through your quads. Squeeze through your chest to support the core and make the hold easier.

COMMON FAULTS

- Sagging lower back
- Butt lifted higher than the head and heels
- Improper alignment of shoulders and wrists

PAYOFF This is an unstable variation of plank to amp up the core challenge.

SUPPORTED SIDE
STABILITY BALL PLANK

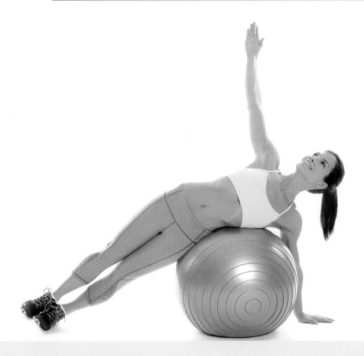

> **SKILL LEVEL:** Intermediate

> **MODIFICATIONS:** Can be performed with ball braced against a stable surface or the feet can be split (for more support)

In this variation of side plank, you will maintain a static hold with the stability ball placed under the side body.

KEY PERFORMANCE POINTS

- Position the stability ball under your rib cage and hips, on the side of your body facing the floor.
- Place the working hand on the floor directly underneath your shoulder, and press into your palm to stabilize the shoulder joint.
- Stack your hips and feet on top of one another to create a straight line from your head to your heels.

COMMON FAULTS

- Hips rotated forward or backward
- Hand placement not in alignment with the shoulder

PAYOFF This exercise targets the obliques and strengthens the shoulder stabilizers.

FOREARM

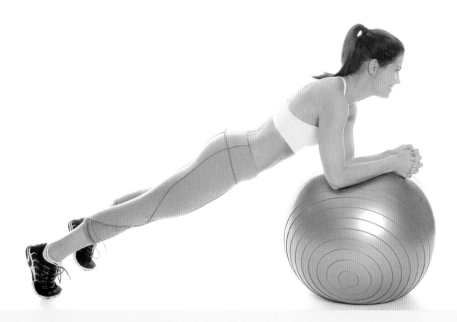

> **SKILL LEVEL: Intermediate**

> **MODIFICATION: Place stability ball against a stable service such as a wall (for more support)**

This is an unstable forearm plank variation performed with forearms on the stability ball and feet on the floor as you maintain a static hold.

KEY PERFORMANCE POINTS

- Place your forearms on the stability ball and feet on the floor; maintain a straight body position from your head to your heels.
- Stack your shoulders directly over your elbows, and press your forearms into the stability ball to support your shoulders.
- Maintain a tight core while squeezing through your quads and chest.

COMMON FAULTS

- Sagging lower back
- Butt lifted higher than the head and heels
- Improper alignment of shoulders and elbows

PAYOFF Get ready to shake as you test your endurance in this challenging plank.

SIDE FOREARM
STABILITY BALL PLANK

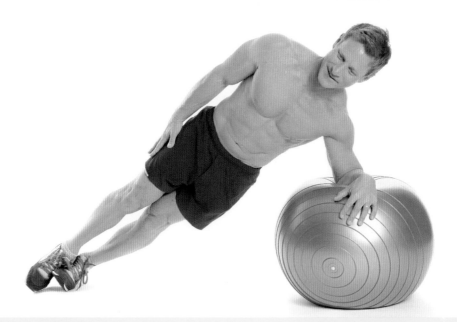

> **SKILL LEVEL: Intermediate**

> **MODIFICATIONS: Can be performed with ball braced against a stable surface or the feet can be split (for more support)**

Here you will maintain a static hold in side forearm plank with the forearm on a stability ball.

KEY PERFORMANCE POINTS

- Place your elbow in the center of the stability ball; Align your shoulder directly over your elbow.

- Press your forearm into the stability ball to support the shoulder joint.

- Stack your hips and feet on top of one another to create a straight line from your head to your heels; actively lift the side of your body up as high as possible.

COMMON FAULTS

- Side body sagging

- Hips rotated forward or backward

- Elbow placement not in line with shoulder

PAYOFF This plank builds strong shoulders while whittling away at the waist.

BALANCING

STABILITY BALL PLANK

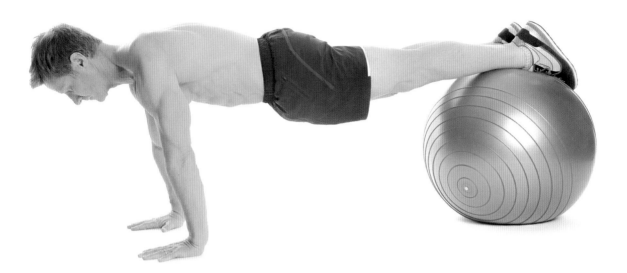

> **SKILL LEVEL: Intermediate**

> **MODIFICATION: Place stability ball against a stable service such as a wall (for more support)**

Here you will maintain a static hold in full plank while balancing with shins and tops of feet on the stability ball and hands on the floor.

KEY PERFORMANCE POINTS

- Stack your shoulders directly over your wrists; place the tops of your feet and shins on the stability ball.
- Maintain a straight body position from your head to your heels and a tight core while squeezing through your quads and chest to support the core and make the hold easier.

COMMON FAULTS

- Sagging lower back
- Butt lifted higher than the head and heels
- Improper alignment of shoulders and wrists

PAYOFF This is a total body workout because the body works to stabilize and hold the plank.

KNEE TUCKS

STABILITY BALL PLANK

> **SKILL LEVEL: Intermediate**

> **MODIFICATION: None**

This variation introduces movement to the stability ball plank with the addition of knee tucks. Begin in a stability ball balancing plank, and then move through reps of drawing the knees in towards the chest and pushing back to full plank.

KEY PERFORMANCE POINTS

- Stack your shoulders directly over your wrists, and place the tops of your feet and shins on the stability ball.
- Maintain a tight core while drawing your knees into your chest and contracting your abdomen.

COMMON FAULTS

- Improper alignment of shoulders and wrists
- Ball only placed on tops of the feet and not on shins

PAYOFF This variation adds a crunch to your plank to tone your abs.

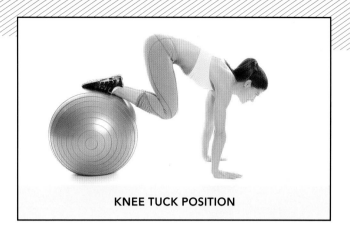

KNEE TUCK POSITION

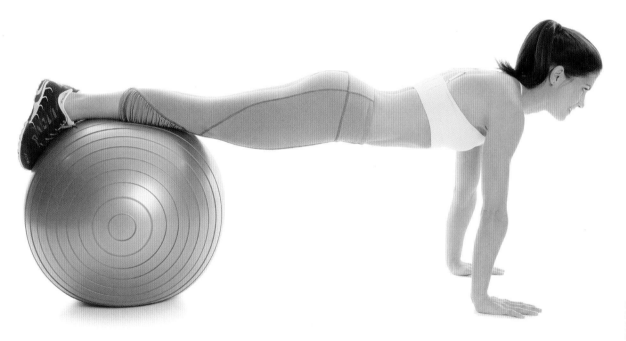

WALKS

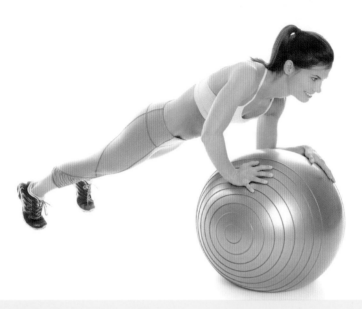

> **SKILL LEVEL: Intermediate**

> **MODIFICATION: Place the stability ball against a stable surface such as a wall (for more support)**

This is the unstable variation of the plank walks performed in the first chapter (see page 26). Adding the stability ball makes the movement much harder.

KEY PERFORMANCE POINTS

- Get into a full plank with a straight body position from your head to your heels with your shoulders stacked over your wrists and firmly plant your palms on either side of the stability ball.

- Walk your hands from full plank to forearm plank and back up to full plank again on the stability ball. Repeat on the other side for one rep.

- Keep your hips square to the floor as you perform the walk.

COMMON FAULTS

- Sagging lower back

- One hip lifted higher than the other during the walking movement

- Improper alignment of your shoulders, elbows, and wrists

PAYOFF Alternate full plank and forearm plank on the stability ball to build a flat belly.

BALANCING SIDE FOREARM

STABILITY BALL PLANK

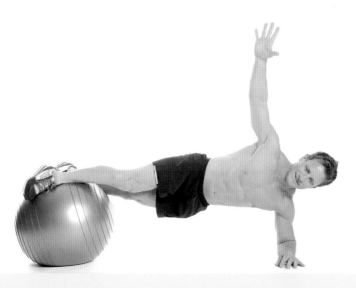

> **SKILL LEVEL: Advanced**

> **MODIFICATION: Place stability ball against a stable service such as a wall (for more support)**

This variation of side plank requires tons of balance, coordination, and core control as you maintain a static hold in side forearm plank with feet on the stability ball.

KEY PERFORMANCE POINTS

- Place your feet on the stability ball; split your feet so that each foot is on the stability ball.

- Place the working hand on the floor directly underneath your shoulder, and press into your palm to stabilize the shoulder joint.

- Stack your hips on top of one another to create a straight line from your head to your heels, and drive through your side to lift your hips toward the ceiling.

COMMON FAULTS

- Hips rotated forward or backward

- Hand placement not in alignment with the shoulder

- Improper foot positioning

PAYOFF This plank challenges your balance, coordination, and strength.

STIR THE POT
STABILITY BALL PLANK

> **SKILL LEVEL: Intermediate**

> **MODIFICATION: None**

This variation begins in a stability ball forearm plank and then adds a stirring motion with the elbows. The movement of the ball creates an even tougher forearm plank challenge. Be sure to stir clockwise and counter-clockwise.

KEY PERFORMANCE POINTS

- Get into a forearm plank on the stability ball; maintain a straight body position from your head to your heels.
- Press your forearms into the stability ball to support the shoulder joint; squeeze through your quads to support your core and keep your hips square.
- Perform a stirring motion with your elbows, making small circles to your left and to your right.

COMMON FAULTS

- Sagging lower back
- Hips rotated out of alignment with one hip lifted higher

PAYOFF This exercise works the shoulders, biceps, triceps, and back as it tones the core.

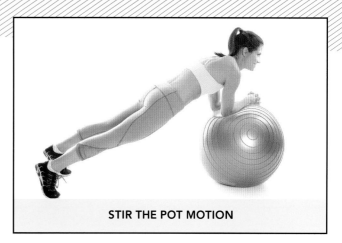

STIR THE POT MOTION

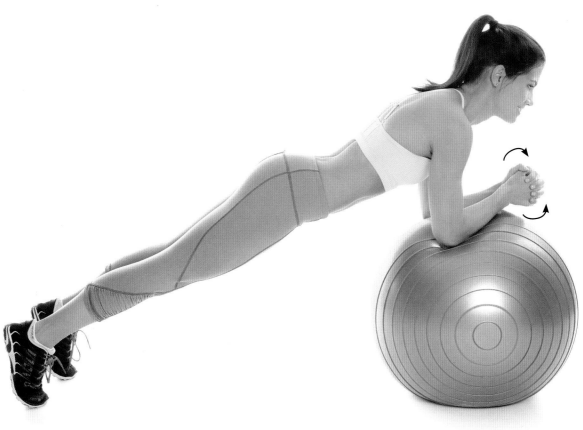

REVERSE

STABILITY BALL PLANK

> **SKILL LEVEL: Beginner**

> **MODIFICATION: Can be performed with bent knees in a table position (to make it easier)**

In this variation, you're flipping over onto the back in this restorative variation of reverse plank.

KEY PERFORMANCE POINTS

- Recline back onto the stability ball, positioning the ball underneath your shoulder blades so it supports your head and neck.
- Press into your feet and squeeze your gluteus and quads to lift your hips.
- Allow your arms to fall out in a T–shape to open your chest and stretch your shoulders.

COMMON FAULTS

- Sagging hips
- Lifted toes
- Stability ball does not properly support your head and neck

PAYOFF This plank strengthens and tones the butt while also opening the front side of the body.

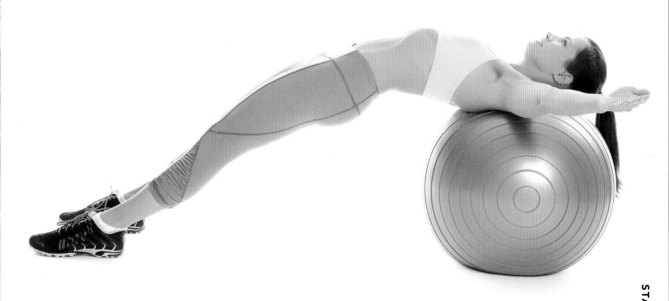

MODIFICATION OF REVERSE PLANK

CHAPTER SIX

BOSU TRAINER PLANKS

ADVANCE YOUR STABILITY AND TARGET SUPPORTING MUSCLES

The second unstable surface that you will work with is the BOSU Trainer. This is the big, blue half circle that you've likely seen around the gym. BOSU is short for "Both Sides Utilized." One of the best features of this piece of the equipment is the ability to scale the intensity based on what side of the ball you work with.

The benefits of the BOSU Trainer are similar to those of the stability ball. Working on an unstable surface requires all the muscles of the core to work harder to stabilize and support the body. Performing plank variations on the BOSU will result in enhanced balance and coordination in addition to a stronger core.

You should be able to perform a solid full plank before moving on to the BOSU.

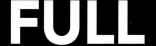

FULL

BOSU TRAINER PLANK

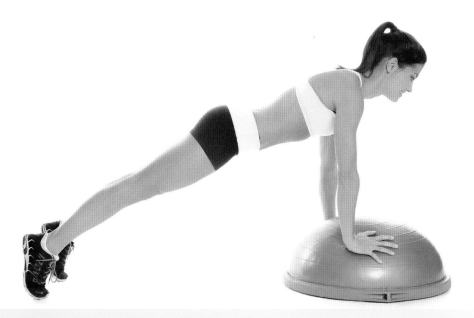

> **SKILL LEVEL: Beginner**

> **MODIFICATIONS: Can be performed on knees in full plank or forearm plank (to make it easier)**

In the BOSU full plank, you will maintain a static hold in a full plank position, with your hands on the BOSU, flat-side down, and feet on the floor.

KEY PERFORMANCE POINTS

- Stack your shoulders directly over your wrists. Place your hands on either side of the ball and press into your palms.

- Maintain a straight body position from your head to your heels, as well as a tight core, while squeezing through your quads and chest to support the core (to make the hold easier).

COMMON FAULTS

- Sagging lower back
- Butt lifted higher than the head and heels
- Improper alignment of shoulders and wrists

PAYOFF This plank sculpts the entire abdominal wall and builds upper body strength.

FLIPPED

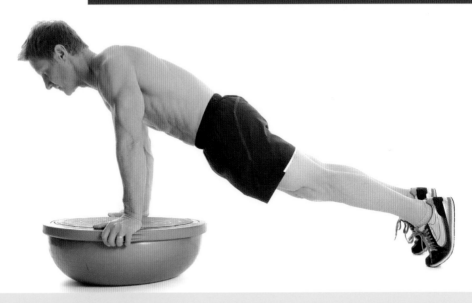

> **SKILL LEVEL:** Intermediate

> **MODIFICATIONS:** Can be performed on knees or in full plank or forearm plank (to make it easier)

In the flipped BOSU plank, you will maintain a static hold in a full plank position, with your hands on the BOSU, ball-side down, and feet on the floor. You can add a little rocking motion back and forth or side to side to make this harder.

KEY PERFORMANCE POINTS

- Stack your shoulders directly over your wrists. Place your hands on the handles of the BOSU.
- Maintain a straight body position from your head to your heels, as well as a tight core, while squeezing through your quads and chest to support the core (to make the hold easier).

COMMON FAULTS

- Sagging lower back
- Butt lifted higher than the head and heels
- Improper alignment of shoulders and wrists

PAYOFF This plank stabilizes the shoulders and strengthens the core.

WALKS

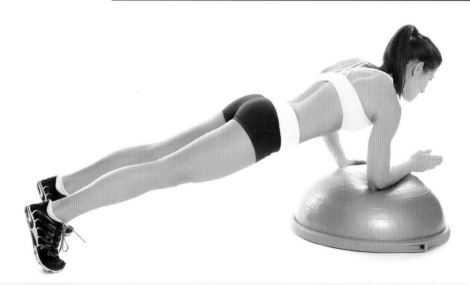

> **SKILL LEVEL: Intermediate**

> **MODIFICATION: Can be performed on the knees (to make it easier)**

This is another unstable variation of the plank walks you did in the first chapter (see page 26). The BOSU will give you a little more support than the stability ball.

KEY PERFORMANCE POINTS

- Place the BOSU ball flat-side down.

- Maintain a straight body position from your head through your heels with your shoulders stacked over your wrists or elbows throughout the movement.

- Keep your hips square to the floor as you walk from palms to forearms and back up to palms again.

COMMON FAULTS

- Sagging lower back

- One hip lifted higher than the other during the walking movement

- Improper alignment of your shoulders, elbows, and wrists

PAYOFF In this exercise, movement plus unstable surfaces equals excellent results.

SIDE FOREARM
BOSU TRAINER PLANK

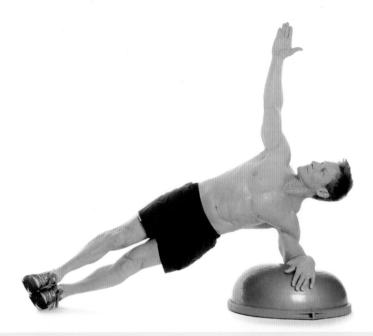

> **SKILL LEVEL: Intermediate**

> **MODIFICATION: Bring the bottom knee to the floor (for more stability)**

Here you will maintain a static hold in side forearm plank, with the forearm on a BOSU Trainer.

KEY PERFORMANCE POINTS

- Place your elbow in the center of the BOSU; align your shoulder directly over your elbow.
- Press your forearm into the BOSU to support the shoulder joint.
- Stack your hips and feet on top of one another to create a straight line from your head to your heels, and actively lift the side of your body up as high as possible.

COMMON FAULTS

- Side body sagging
- Hips rotated forward or backward
- Elbow placement not in line with shoulder

PAYOFF This plank uses long holds to slim the waist.

SIDE FOREARM WITH KNEE CRUNCHES

BOSU TRAINER PLANK

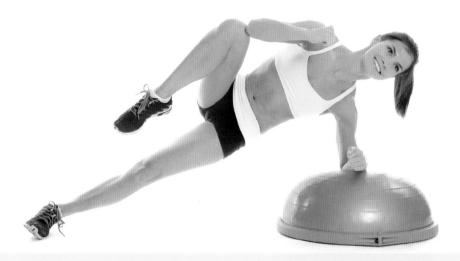

> **SKILL LEVEL: Intermediate**

> **MODIFICATION: Bring the bottom knee to the floor (for more stability)**

Adding the BOSU to your knee crunch side plank challenges shoulder stabilization to hold the side plank, while also adding movement through knee crunches.

KEY PERFORMANCE POINTS

- Place your elbow in the center of the BOSU; press into your forearm to lift through the side of your body.
- Stack your hips and feet on top of one another to create a straight line from your head to your heels.
- Lift your top leg up a few inches and then draw that knee and lifted arm into your chest, and then reach both away.

COMMON FAULTS

- Side body sagging
- Hips and shoulders rotated forward or backward
- Hand placement not in line with shoulder

PAYOFF This plank creates chiseled abs and a strong side body.

CHAPTER SEVEN

MEDICINE BALL
PLANKS

PERFECT ADVANCED
UNSTABLE SURFACE MOVES

Medicine balls provide another unstable surface for you to work on. While they are much smaller than the stability ball and BOSU Trainer, don't let their small size fool you. Performing planks on the medicine ball is a fast track to a strong, stable shoulder and a tight core.

This is a challenging unstable surface, so a strong full plank is a must before progressing to the medicine ball. Medicine balls come in a variety of weights, but, for the purpose of the planks in this book, any weight is fine since none of these variations require lifting the medicine balls from the floor.

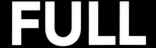

FULL

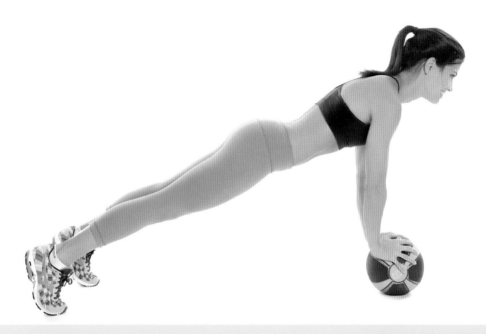

> **SKILL LEVEL: Intermediate**

> **MODIFICATION: Can be performed on knees (to make it easier)**

For the medicine ball full plank, you will maintain a static hold in a full plank position, with your hands on the medicine ball and feet on the floor.

KEY PERFORMANCE POINTS

- Stack your shoulders directly over your wrists. Place your hands on either side of the medicine ball and press into your palms.
- Maintain a straight body position from your head to your heels with feet hip distance apart.
- Maintain a tight core while squeezing through your quads and chest to support the core (to make the hold easier).

COMMON FAULTS

- Sagging lower back
- Butt lifted higher than the head and heels
- Improper alignment of shoulders and wrists

PAYOFF This exercise builds balance and coordination.

DOUBLE
MEDICINE BALL PLANK

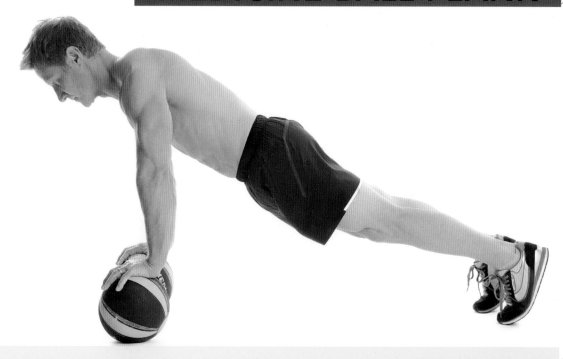

> **SKILL LEVEL: Advanced**

> **MODIFICATION: Can be performed on knees (to make it easier)**

You're kicking it up a notch in this variation by placing your hands on two medicine balls instead of one, which gives you an extra balance and stability challenge. Maintain a static hold.

KEY PERFORMANCE POINTS

- Stack your shoulders directly over your wrists. Place two medicine balls shoulder width apart, and place your hands in the center of each ball. Press into your palms.

- Maintain a straight body position from your head to your heels, with your feet hip width apart.

- Maintain a tight core while squeezing through your quads and chest to support the core (to make the hold easier).

COMMON FAULTS

- Sagging lower back

- Butt lifted higher than the head and heels

- Improper alignment of shoulders and wrists

PAYOFF This plank is a major stability challenge.

ROLLING
MEDICINE BALL PLANK

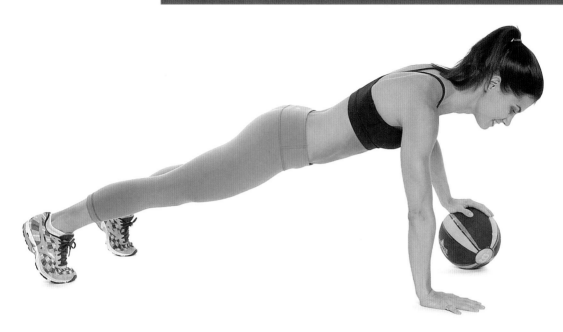

> **SKILL LEVEL: Intermediate**

> **MODIFICATION: Can be performed on knees (to make it easier)**

In this medicine ball plank variation, you will place the medicine ball under one hand and then roll it across the body and switch hands. Each pass back and forth is one rep.

KEY PERFORMANCE POINTS

- Stack your shoulders over your wrists. Place one palm on the medicine ball and the other on the floor.

- Maintain a straight body position from your head to your heels, with your feet hip width apart as you pass the medicine ball from one hand to the other.

- Maintain a tight core while squeezing through your quads and chest to support the core (to make the hold easier).

COMMON FAULTS

- Sagging lower back

- Butt lifted higher than the head and heels

- Improper alignment of shoulders and wrists

PAYOFF This plank builds balance and coordination.

LEG LIFT

MEDICINE BALL PLANK

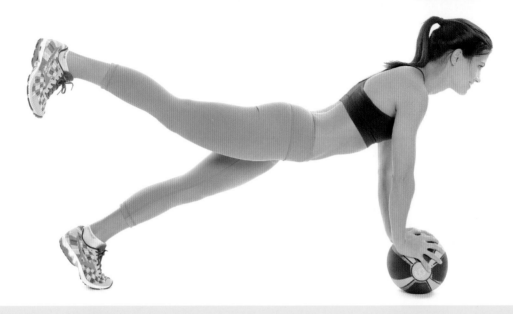

> **SKILL LEVEL: Intermediate**

> **MODIFICATION: Can be performed in a static hold with a leg lift instead of pulsing (to make it easier)**

In this variation of medicine ball full plank, one leg will lift off of the ground and pulse while holding the plank.

KEY PERFORMANCE POINTS

- Stack your shoulders over your wrists. Place your hands on either side of the medicine ball and press into your palms.
- Maintain a straight body position from your head to your heels, with one leg lifting up and pulsing.
- Maintain a tight core while squeezing through your quads and chest to support the core (to make the hold easier).

COMMON FAULTS

- Sagging lower back
- Working leg hip lifted higher than the grounded leg hip
- Improper alignment of shoulders and wrists

PAYOFF This variation tightens the tummy as it strengthens the hip flexors.

CHEETAH

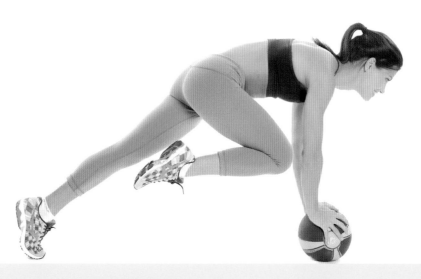

> **SKILL LEVEL: Intermediate**

> **MODIFICATION: Drop to one knee (for more stability)**

In this variation of medicine ball full plank, one leg will lift and move through a range of motion, where it will draw into the chest and then push away.

KEY PERFORMANCE POINTS

- Stack your shoulders directly over your wrists. Place your hands on either side of the medicine ball, and press into your palms.

- Maintain a straight body position from your head to your heels, with one leg lifted up. Draw your knee of the lifted leg into your chest, and then press through your heel with your toes pointing down.

- Maintain a tight core while squeezing through your quads and chest to support the core (to make the hold easier).

- For an extra kick, twist your knee to the opposite tricep, or bring your knee to the outside of your elbow.

COMMON FAULTS

- Shin not lifted high enough during the cheetah motion

- Working leg hip lifted higher than the grounded leg hip

- Improper alignment of shoulders and wrists

PAYOFF This variation combines a crunch and a plank to tighten the core.

SIDE

MEDICINE BALL PLANK

> **SKILL LEVEL: Advanced**

> **MODIFICATION: Bring the bottom knee to the floor (for more stability)**

Here you will maintain a static hold in side plank while balancing with one hand on a medicine ball.

KEY PERFORMANCE POINTS

- Place your palm in the center of the medicine ball; align your shoulder directly over your palm.
- Press your palm firmly into the medicine ball to support your shoulder joint.
- Stack your hips and feet on top of one another to create a straight line from your head to your heels, and actively lift the side of your body up as high as possible.

COMMON FAULTS

- Side body sagging
- Hips rotated forward or backward
- Elbow placement not in line with shoulder

PAYOFF This exercise is the ultimate in shoulder stabilization and body control.

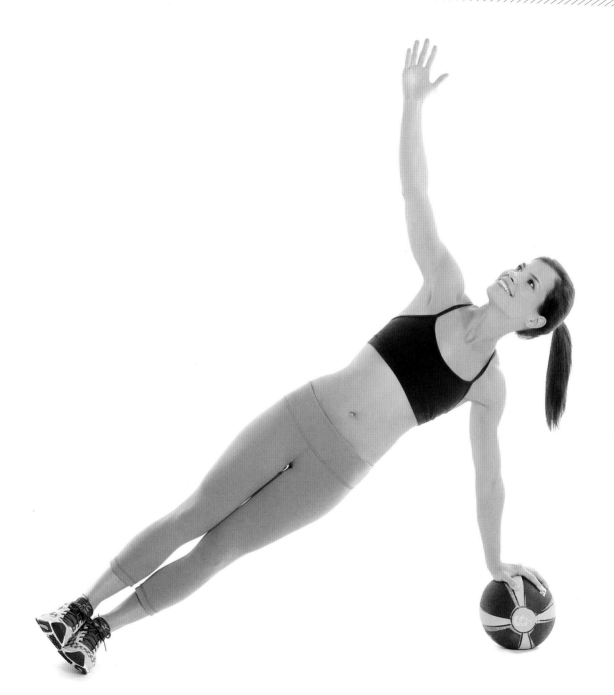

PART THREE

PLANKS
WITH EQUIPMENT + PLYOMETRIC PLANKS

The planks in this section are exercise-based and focus on using weights, gliding disks, and plyometric movements to challenge the body in new ways. They also give you additional toning benefits in other muscle groups while you strengthen the core.

A well-rounded fitness routine should include strength, cardiovascular, core, flexibility, and balance training. It's efficient and effective to combine these elements whenever possible.

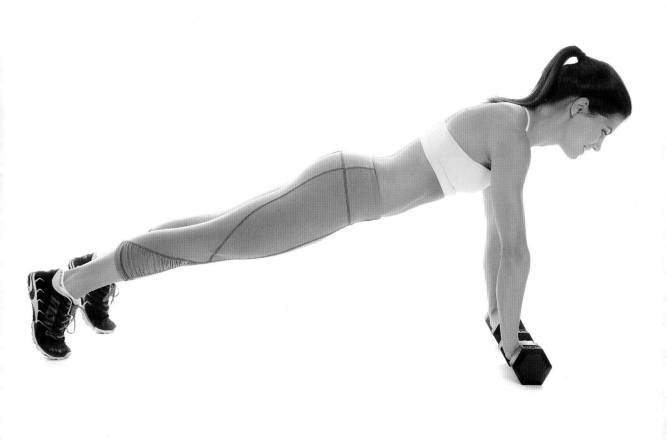

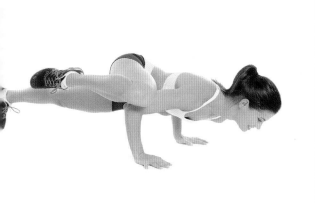

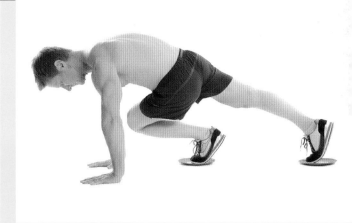

CHAPTER EIGHT

PLANKS

WITH WEIGHTS

STRENGTH TRAINING FOR A STRONG CORE AND SCULPTED BODY

The planks in this chapter incorporate dumbbells and plates to add strength training and total body toning to our core work. Here you'll find both weighted plank variations and traditional dumbbell exercises performed while holding a plank or a supported reverse plank position on a stability ball.

DUMBBELL PUNCH

PLANK WITH WEIGHTS

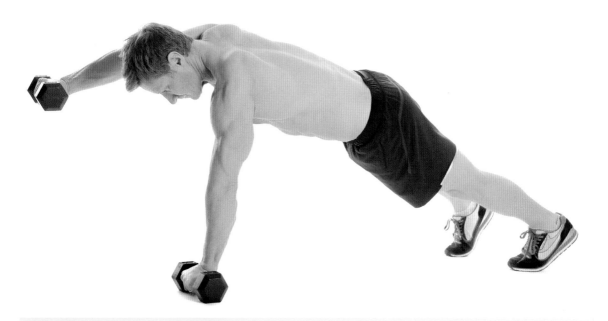

> **SKILL LEVEL: Intermediate**

> **MODIFICATION: Can be performed on knees (to make it easier)**

This exercise combines a full plank hold with dumbbell front punches.

KEY PERFORMANCE POINTS

- Place your hands on two dumbbells and get into a full plank position.

- Maintain a straight body position from your head to your heels with your feet wider than your hips to help keep the hips square throughout the movement.

- Draw one dumbbell up toward your shoulder and punch it straight out in front of you, with your knuckles facing the ceiling and your bicep by your ear. Alternate your right and left sides.

COMMON FAULTS

- Sagging lower back

- Butt lifted higher than the head and heels on the working side

- Punching arm not lifted in line with your head

PAYOFF This plank creates a rock solid shoulder.

DUMBBELL ROWS

PLANK WITH WEIGHTS

> **SKILL LEVEL: Intermediate**

> **MODIFICATION: Can be performed on knees (to make it easier)**

This exercise combines a full plank hold with weighted rows to work the core and the upper back.

KEY PERFORMANCE POINTS

- Place your hands on two dumbbells and get into a full plank position.
- Maintain a straight body position from your head to your heels, with your feet hip width apart.
- Draw one elbow back and toward the ceiling as you squeeze through your shoulder blade. Alternate right and left sides.
- For an additional benefit, add a push-up after each rep.

COMMON FAULTS

- Sagging lower back
- Butt lifted higher than the head and heels on the working side
- Improper alignment of shoulders and wrists

PAYOFF This plank builds beautiful back muscles.

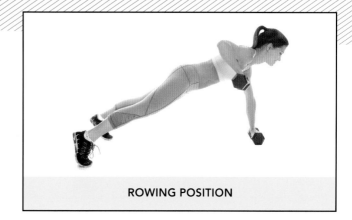

ROWING POSITION

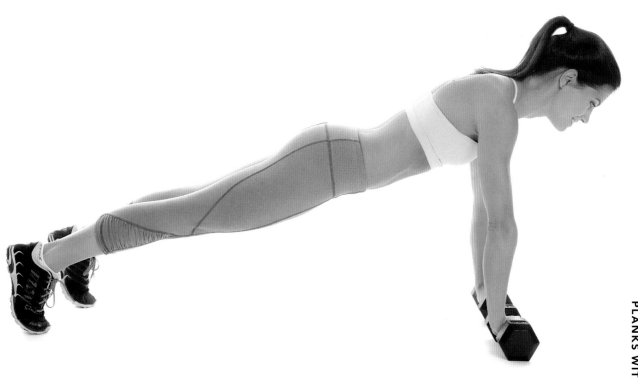

DUMBBELL TRICEP KICKBACKS

PLANK WITH WEIGHTS

> **SKILL LEVEL: Intermediate**

> **MODIFICATION: Can be performed on knees (to make it easier)**

This exercise combines a full plank hold with weighted kickbacks to work the core and the triceps.

KEY PERFORMANCE POINTS

- Place your hands on two dumbbells and get into a full plank position.
- Maintain a straight body position from your head to your heels, with your feet hip width apart.
- Draw one elbow up toward the ceiling, creating a 90-degree bend, and then straighten your elbow by pressing the dumbbell behind you. Return to a 90-degree bend to complete the kickback movement.
- Keep your elbow glued to the side of your body, and squeeze the tricep at the top of the movement.

COMMON FAULTS

- Sagging lower back
- Butt lifted higher than the head and heels on the working side
- Elbow not tucked into the side body while performing the kickback

PAYOFF This exercise defines the triceps.

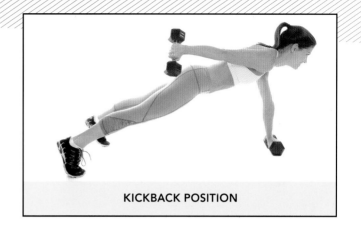

KICKBACK POSITION

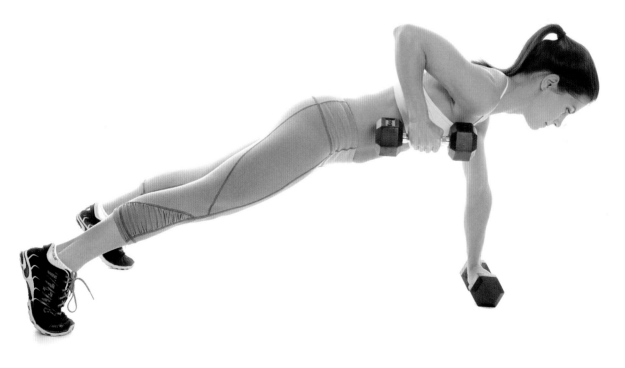

FULL

PLANK WITH WEIGHTS

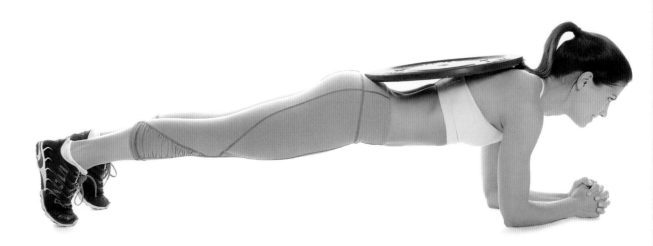

> **SKILL LEVEL: Intermediate**

> **MODIFICATION: Can be performed on knees (to make it easier)**

Here you will maintain a static hold in full or forearm plank, with a weighted plate placed on the back.

KEY PERFORMANCE POINTS

- Maintain a straight body position from your head through your heels with your gaze down to the floor.
- Stack your shoulders directly over your wrists, and plant your palms firmly on the floor.
- Place the plate on your back.
- Maintain a tight core while squeezing through your quads and chest to support the core (to make the hold easier).

COMMON FAULTS

- Sagging lower back
- Butt lifted higher than your head and your heels
- Improper alignment of shoulders and wrists

PAYOFF This plank, with the extra weighted plate, builds total body strength.

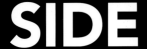

SIDE

PLANK WITH WEIGHTS

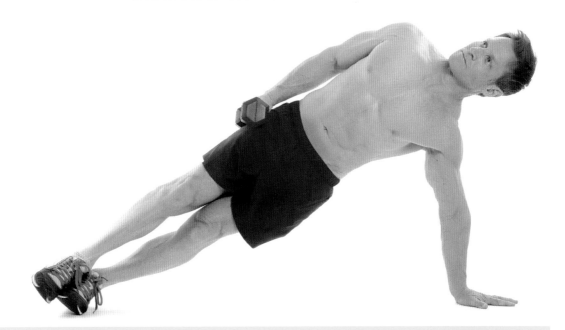

> **SKILL LEVEL: Intermediate**

> **MODIFICATION: Ground one knee down to the floor (to make it easier)**

Maintain a static hold in a full side plank or forearm side plank while holding a dumbbell against the side body.

KEY PERFORMANCE POINTS

- Place the working hand on the floor directly underneath your shoulder, and press into your palm to stabilize the shoulder joint.
- Stack your hips and feet on top of one another to create a straight line from your head to your heels.
- Rest a dumbbell against the lifted side body near your hips.

COMMON FAULTS

- Side body sagging
- Hips rotated forward or backward
- Hand not in line with the shoulder

PAYOFF This plank weighs down your side plank to cut down your waist.

STAR SIDE
PLANK WITH WEIGHTS

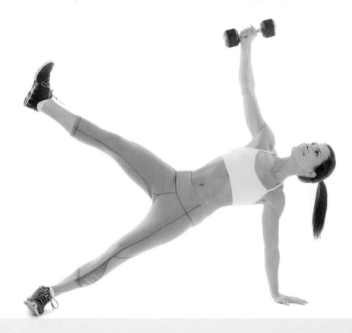

> **SKILL LEVEL: Advanced**

> **MODIFICATION: Ground one knee down to the floor (to make it easier)**

Here you will maintain a static hold in a full side plank or forearm side plank while holding a dumbbell straight up in the air and lifting a leg.

KEY PERFORMANCE POINTS

- Place the working hand on the floor directly underneath your shoulder; press into your palm to stabilize your shoulder joint.
- Stack your hips and feet on top of one another to create a straight line from your head to your heels.
- Raise a dumbbell in line with the shoulder straight overhead, and lift your top leg to form a star shape.

COMMON FAULTS

- Side body sagging
- Hips rotated forward or backward
- Hand not in line with the shoulder

PAYOFF This plank builds balance, core strength, and shoulder stabilization.

STABILITY BALL CHEST PRESS

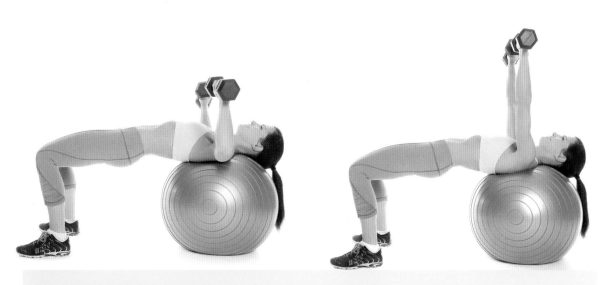

> **SKILL LEVEL: Beginner**

> **MODIFICATION: None**

This exercise combines a supported hold in reverse table on the stability ball with reps of chest presses with dumbbells.

KEY PERFORMANCE POINTS

- Recline back onto the stability ball, positioning the ball underneath your shoulder blades to support your head and neck.

- Press into your feet and squeeze your gluteus and quads to lift your hips.

- Start with the dumbbells horizontally stacked over your shoulders. Draw your elbows down in line with your shoulder, and then engage through your chest to press back up.

COMMON FAULTS

- Sagging hips

- Insufficient support of your head and neck from the stability ball

- Lifted toes

PAYOFF This is a two-for-one gluteus toner and chest developer.

STABILITY BALL CHEST FLY

PLANK WITH WEIGHTS

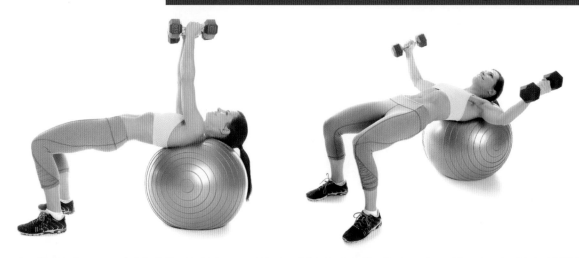

> **SKILL LEVEL: Beginner**

> **MODIFICATION: None**

This exercise combines a supported hold in reverse table on the stability ball with reps of chest fly with dumbbells.

KEY PERFORMANCE POINTS

- Recline back onto the stability ball, positioning the ball underneath your shoulder blades to support your head and neck.

- Press into your feet and squeeze your gluteus and quads to lift your hips.

- Start with dumbbells stacked vertically over your shoulders with your palms facing inward. With slightly bent elbows, draw your elbows down until they are in line with your shoulders. Engage through your chest to bring them back together. Imagine that you are squeezing a big beach ball with your arms.

COMMON FAULTS

- Sagging hips
- Insufficient support of your head and neck from the stability ball
- Lifted toes

PAYOFF This is a two-for-one gluteus toner and chest developer.

STABILITY BALL OVERHEAD EXTENSION

PLANK WITH WEIGHTS

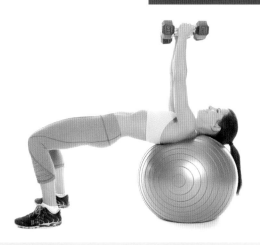 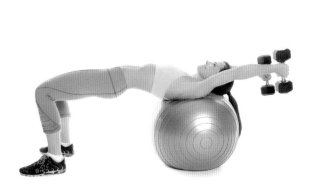

> **SKILL LEVEL:** Beginner

> **MODIFICATION:** None

This exercise combines a supported hold in reverse table on the stability ball with reps of overhead extension with dumbbells.

KEY PERFORMANCE POINTS

- Recline back onto stability ball, positioning the ball underneath your shoulder blades to support your head and neck.

- Press into your feet, and squeeze your gluteus and quads to lift your hips.

- Start with the dumbbells vertically stacked over your shoulders. With straight arms, extend the dumbbells over your head until your biceps are in line with your ear.

- Engage through your core and your lats to bring the dumbbells back to the starting position.

COMMON FAULTS

- Sagging hips
- Insufficient support of your head and neck from the stability ball
- Bent elbows

PAYOFF This exercise produces a strong and sexy back.

FOREARM PLANK PLATE PUSH + PULL

PLANK WITH WEIGHTS

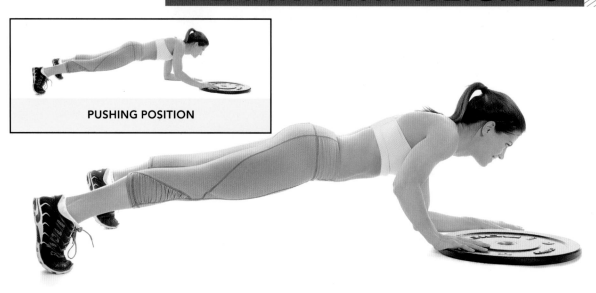

PUSHING POSITION

> **SKILL LEVEL: Intermediate**

> **MODIFICATION: Drop down to knees (to make it easier)**

This exercise combines a static hold in a forearm plank with pushing and pulling a weighted plate with one hand.

KEY PERFORMANCE POINTS

- Get into a forearm plank and maintain a straight line from your head to your heels.
- Squeeze through your quads to keep your hips square and to support your core.
- Place a weighted plate under one hand, and alternate pushing it forward and then pulling it back to you.

COMMON FAULTS

- Sagging lower back
- One hip lifted higher than the other

PAYOFF This exercise works the shoulders, abs, and back with one move.

CHAPTER NINE

PLYOMETRIC
PLANKS

INCREASE YOUR HEART RATE FOR KILLER CARDIO

Get ready to drive your heart rate up with these plyometric plank variations. In addition to blasting fat and calories, including plyometric exercises in your training routine increases muscular power and explosiveness while also building endurance.

Plyometrics use movements such as jumping and bounding in fast succession to move the muscles through a cycle of lengthening (eccentric contraction) and shortening (concentric contraction). Pairing these movements together trains your body to decrease the time between the eccentric and concentric contractions and results in increased neuromuscular control, power, and speed. Another benefit of plyometric exercises is that there is no special equipment needed—just your own body weight and clear floor space.

The plank variations that follow are great on their own but also work well when alternated with static planks to create a core training workout that keeps the heart rate elevated.

LATERAL HOPPING
PLYOMETRIC PLANK

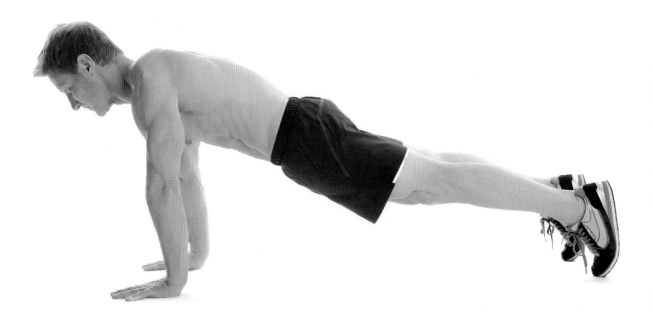

> **SKILL LEVEL: Intermediate**

> **MODIFICATION: Hop the feet only or hands only, instead of both at the same time (to make it easier)**

In this plyometric plank, you alternate performing small hops to the right and left while maintaining a full plank position.

KEY PERFORMANCE POINTS

- Get into a full plank position with your hands under your shoulders and a straight line from your head to your heels.

- Slightly bend your knees and push into your palms to hop your body from side to side, maintaining your full plank position the entire time.

- Be sure to land gently with slightly bent elbows and softened joints to absorb the impact.

COMMON FAULTS

- Sagging lower back
- Locked out joints

PAYOFF This exercise blasts calories and builds explosive strength.

SKI JUMP

PLYOMETRIC PLANK

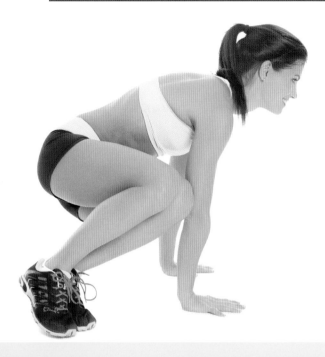

> **SKILL LEVEL: Intermediate**

> **MODIFICATION: None**

This plyometric plank requires you to jump the feet from full plank to the outside of the elbows and back to the full plank.

KEY PERFORMANCE POINTS

- Get into a full plank position with your hands under your shoulders and a straight line from your head to your heels.

- Slightly bend your knees and jump to the outside of your elbows, landing in a deep squat position with your knees outside of your elbows.

- Jump back to full plank position; land with slightly bent elbows and softened joints to absorb shock. Alternate your right and left sides.

COMMON FAULTS

- Locked out joints

- Knees do not get to the outside of your elbows

PAYOFF This exercise drives up the heart rate and trims the waist.

PLANK JACKS
PLYOMETRIC PLANK

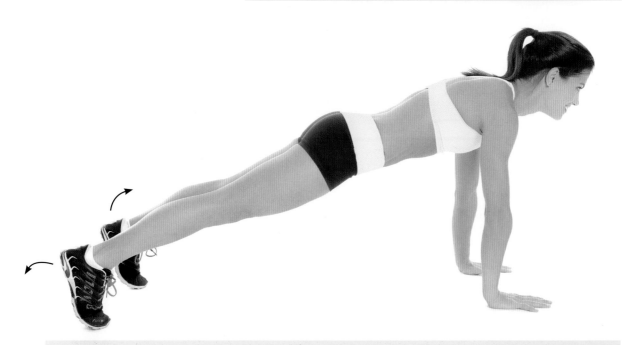

> **SKILL LEVEL: Intermediate**

> **MODIFICATION: None**

In this plyometric plank, you will perform a jumping jack motion with the feet as you hold a static full plank with the upper body.

KEY PERFORMANCE POINTS

- Get into a full plank position with your hands under your shoulders and a straight line from your head to your heels.
- Bring your feet together to touch. Then, hop them wider than your hips, as if you are performing a jumping jack with your lower body.
- Jump your feet back together while keeping your core tight to support the movement.

COMMON FAULTS

- Sagging lower back
- Bent elbows
- Butt lifted higher than the head

PAYOFF This exercise works the inner and outer thighs.

JOGGING

PLYOMETRIC PLANK

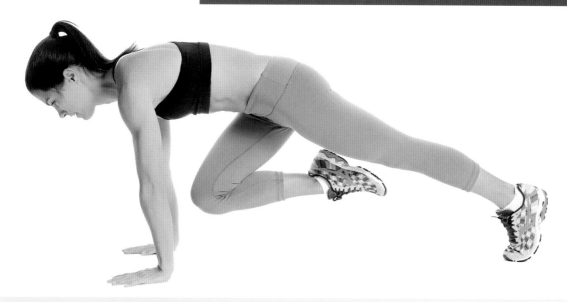

> **SKILL LEVEL: Intermediate**

> **MODIFICATION: None**

In this plyometric plank, the knees alternate jogging into the chest and back to high plank, similar to a jogging motion.

KEY PERFORMANCE POINTS

- Get into a full plank position with your hands under your shoulders and a straight line from your head to your heels.

- Draw one knee into your chest, and then press it back to full plank. Alternate sides and repeat.

- This is a quick movement; you should feel like you are jogging your knees into your chest.

COMMON FAULTS

- Bent elbows

- Excessive rounding of the upper back and a shortened plank position

- Shoulders more forward than wrists

PAYOFF This exercise takes the heart rate through the roof and burns fat.

MOUNTAIN CLIMBER PUSH-UPS

PLYOMETRIC PLANK

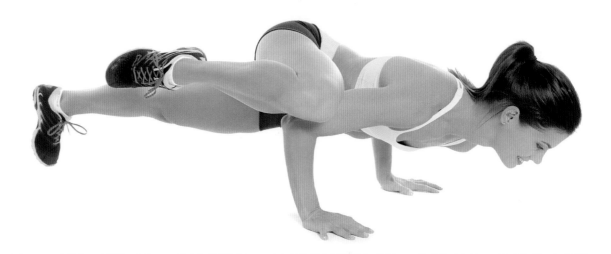

> **SKILL LEVEL: Advanced**

> **MODIFICATION: Skip the push-up (to make it easier)**

In this plyometric plank, you will draw one knee to the outside of the tricep, perform a push-up, and then press back to full plank.

KEY PERFORMANCE POINTS

- Come into a full plank position with your hands under your shoulders and a straight line from your head to your heels.
- Draw your right knee in and toward the outside of your right tricep.
- As you draw your knee in, lower down to a push-up. As you press back up, take your leg back to full plank. Repeat on your left side.

COMMON FAULTS

- Shoulders more forward than the wrists
- Butt lifted higher than the head

PAYOFF This plank tones the upper body and obliques.

FROG JUMP

PLYOMETRIC PLANK

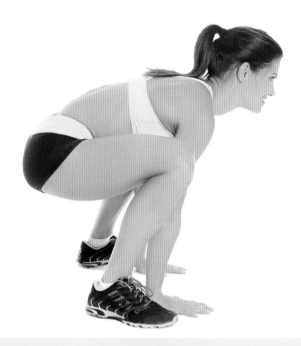

> SKILL LEVEL: Intermediate

> MODIFICATIONS: Step instead of jump (to make it easier) or jump the feet to the inside of the hands instead of the outside (to make it harder)

This plyometric plank requires you to jump the feet from high plank to the outside of the hands and then back to high plank.

KEY PERFORMANCE POINTS

- Get into a full plank position with your hands under your shoulders and a straight line from your head to your heels.
- Slightly bend your knees and explode out of your legs as you jump your feet to the outside of your hands, coming into a deep squat.
- Jump back to a full plank position, and land with slightly bent elbows and softened joints to absorb the shock.

COMMON FAULTS

- Locked out joints
- Feet do not get to the outside of the hands

PAYOFF This exercise builds explosive power and strength.

CHAPTER TEN

GLIDER PLANKS

RECRUIT MULTIPLE MUSCLE GROUPS FOR TOTAL BODY BURN

Glider planks are an effective low-impact solution for core training. With the use of gliding disks, these exercises strengthen the entire body and develop stabilizing muscles. Gliding disks are small and are great to keep on hand for at-home workouts. Don't have a glider? Don't worry—use a paper or plastic plate instead.

Incorporating gliding disks into your core training work is also beneficial because the disks allow you to move through a full range of motion, which in turn increases flexibility and balance. It may take some time to get the hang of gliding planks, but, with practice, you'll soon be able to gracefully perform the plank variations in this chapter.

FOREARM HAND SLIDE

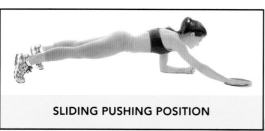

SLIDING PUSHING POSITION

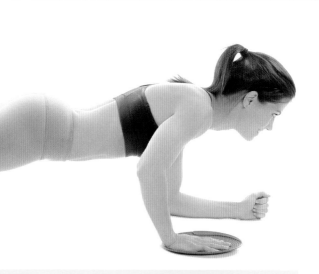

> **SKILL LEVEL: Intermediate**

> **MODIFICATION: Drop down to knees (to make it easier)**

This exercise combines a static hold in the forearm plank with pushing and pulling a gliding disk in front of the body.

KEY PERFORMANCE POINTS

- Get into a forearm plank and maintain a straight line from your head to your heels.
- Squeeze through your quads to keep your hips square and support your core.
- Place a gliding disk under the center of one palm, and alternate pushing it forward and then pulling it back to you. Repeat a set number of reps on each side.

COMMON FAULTS

- Sagging lower back
- One hip lifted higher than the other
- The working arm is not fully extended

PAYOFF This exercise tones the shoulders and builds core control.

FOREARM BODY SAW

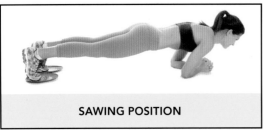

SAWING POSITION

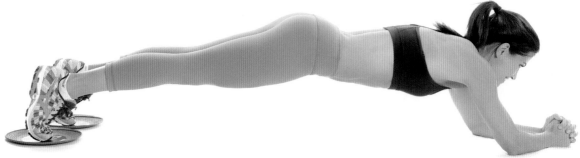

> **SKILL LEVEL: Intermediate**

> **MODIFICATION: None**

This variation requires you to maintain a forearm plank hold as you perform a sawing motion with the body.

KEY PERFORMANCE POINTS

- Place the balls of your feet on the gliding disks. With heels lifted and pressing back, squeeze through your quads to support your core.

- Get into a forearm plank with your elbows under your shoulders, and make a fist with your hands.

- Press into your forearms and draw your shoulders forward of your fist. Then, press into your forearms to draw your shoulders back behind your elbows as you maintain a tight, straight body position.

COMMON FAULTS

- Sagging lower back
- Bent knees
- Improper alignment of shoulders and wrists

PAYOFF This plank works the entire core, shoulders, and lats.

FOREARM HIP ABDUCTION + ADDUCTION

GLIDER PLANK

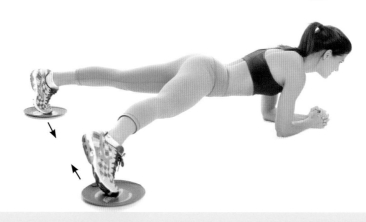

> **SKILL LEVEL: Intermediate**

> **MODIFICATION: Move one leg at a time, alternating legs (to make it easier)**

This gliding plank combines maintaining a forearm plank with moving the lower body through hip abduction and adduction.

KEY PERFORMANCE POINTS

- Place the balls of your feet on the gliding disks. With your heels lifted and pressing back, squeeze through your quads to support your core.
- Get into a forearm plank with your elbows under your shoulders, and make a fist with your hands.
- Slide your feet out wider than your hips by engaging your outer hips, and then slide your feet back to hip width apart by engaging through your inner thighs.

COMMON FAULTS

- Sagging lower back
- Bent knees

PAYOFF This exercise trims and tones the inner and outer thighs.

KNEES TO CHEST
GLIDER PLANK

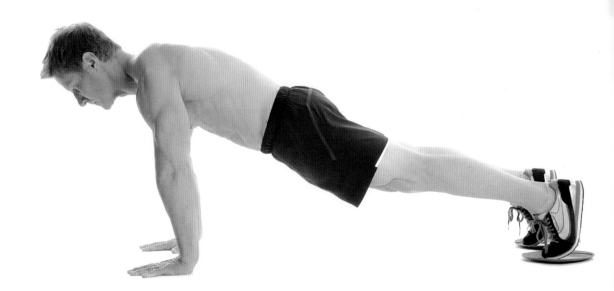

> **SKILL LEVEL: Intermediate**

> **MODIFICATION: Slow it down (to make it easier)**

This gliding plank requires a static hold in full plank as you alternate drawing the knees into the chest in quick jogging-like motions.

KEY PERFORMANCE POINTS

- Place the balls of your feet on the gliding disks, with your heels lifted and pressing back.
- Get into a full plank position with your shoulders stacked over your wrists and a straight line from your head to your heels.
- Draw one knee into your chest, and then press it back to full plank. Alternate sides and repeat.
- This is a quick movement; you should feel like you are jogging your knees into your chest.

COMMON FAULTS

- Shortening of the plank
- Bent elbow

PAYOFF This exercise elevates the heart rate, works the core, and strengthens the hip flexors.

TWISTED KNEE TO CHEST

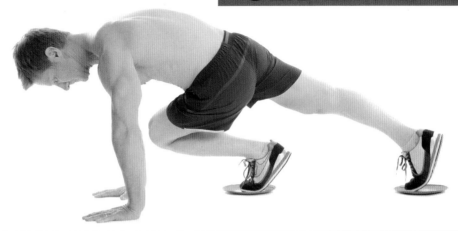

> **SKILL LEVEL:** Intermediate

> **MODIFICATION:** Slow it down (to make it easier) or thread the foot all the way under the arm and straighten out the leg (to make it harder)

This gliding plank requires a static hold in full plank as you alternate drawing the knees to the opposite tricep for an oblique challenge.

KEY PERFORMANCE POINTS

- Place the balls of your feet on gliding disks, with your heels lifted and pressing back.
- Get into a full plank position with your shoulders stacked over your wrists and a straight line from your head to your heels.
- Draw one knee into your chest and toward the opposite tricep, and then press it back to full plank. Alternate sides and repeat.
- This is a quick movement; you should feel like you are jogging your knees back and forth.

COMMON FAULTS

- Shortening of the plank
- Bent elbow

PAYOFF This exercise majorly slims the side body.

GLIDER PLANK

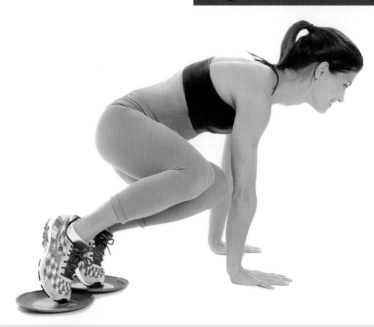

> **SKILL LEVEL: Intermediate**

> **MODIFICATION: None**
> This variation requires the contraction of the abs to pull the knees from full plank to the outside of the elbows.

KEY PERFORMANCE POINTS

- Place the balls of your feet on the glider disks with your heels lifted and pressed back.
- Get into a full plank position with your hands under your shoulders and a straight line from your head to your heels.
- Contract your abdomen, and slide your feet forward, bringing your knees to the outside of your elbows as you get into a deep squat.
- Slide your feet back to the full plank, and repeat on other side.

COMMON FAULTS

- Not getting your knees to the outside of your elbows

PAYOFF This exercise drives up the heart rate and trims the waist.

CRUNCH

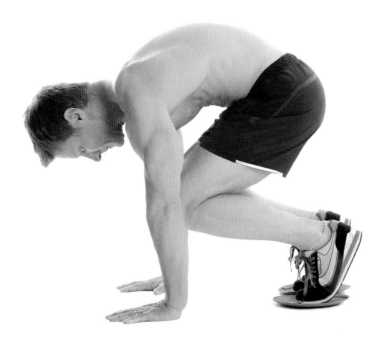

> **SKILL LEVEL: Intermediate**

> **MODIFICATION: None**

Here you use the gliding disks to perform full plank crunches by drawing the knees into the chest at the same time and pressing the feet back out to full plank.

KEY PERFORMANCE POINTS

- Place the balls of your feet on the gliding disks with your heels lifted and pressed back.
- Get into a full plank position with your hands under your shoulders and a straight line from your head to your heels.
- Contract the abdomen, draw your knees into your chest, and slide your feet back to full plank.

COMMON FAULTS

- Bent elbows
- Shoulders more forward than the wrists

PAYOFF This exercise strengthens the hip flexors and creates chiseled abs.

V-UP

> **SKILL LEVEL: Intermediate**

> **MODIFICATION: None**

Use the gliding disks to perform full plank "V-ups" by drawing the feet in toward the hands with straight legs and then pressing back out to the full plank.

KEY PERFORMANCE POINTS

- Place the balls of your feet on the gliding disks with your heels lifted and pressed back.
- Get into a full plank position with your hands under your shoulders and a straight line from your head to your heels.
- Press into your palms, and contract the abdomen as you draw your feet in toward your hands until your body is in a V-shape, with straight legs. Slide back out to the full plank.

COMMON FAULTS

- Bent elbows and knees
- Shoulders more forward than the wrists

PAYOFF This exercise works the rectus abdominis for a six-pack look, and the transverse abdominis to pull the belly in.

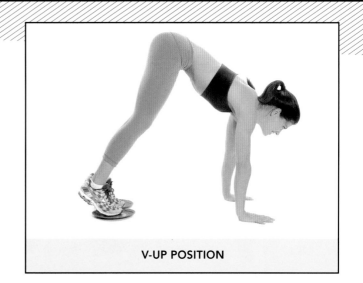

V-UP POSITION

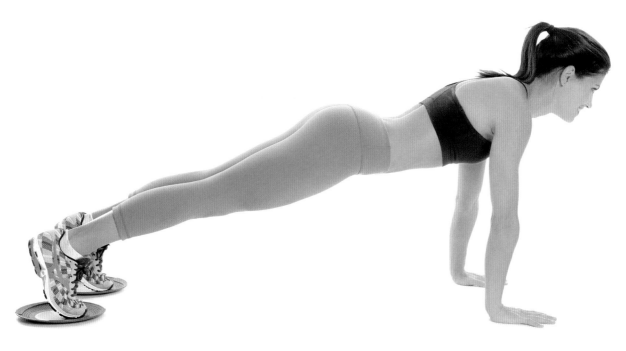

PART FOUR

REVERSE, STRETCHING + EXTRA CREDIT

PLANKS

In this section, it's back to bodyweight planks with no external props to wrap up your plank core training. Start with reverse planks. Flipping the plank is a great way to target and strengthen the muscles in the back of the body. Next, try stretching variations of planks that you can incorporate into your warmup and cooldown to lengthen the muscles.

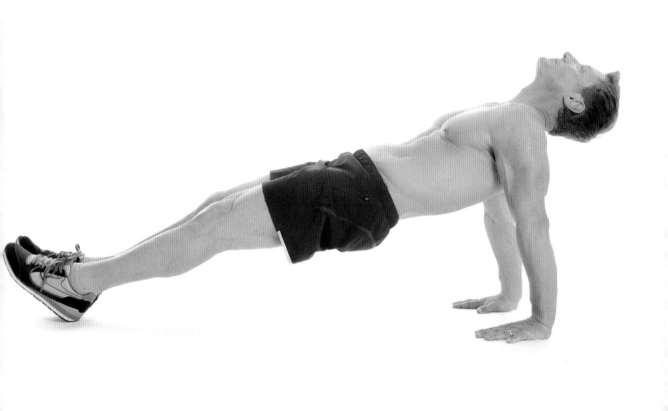

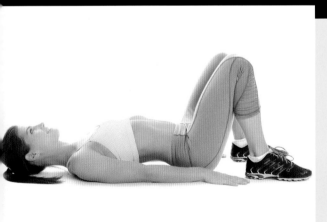

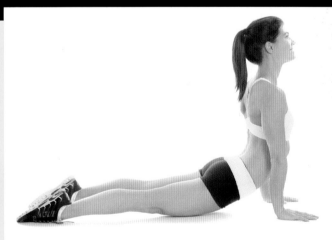

CHAPTER ELEVEN

REVERSE PLANKS

FLIP YOUR PLANK FOR AN INTENSE CORE WORKOUT

When it comes to core training, reverse planks are often forgotten about. Most people focus on working the muscles they can see on the front side of the body. However, reverse planks should be an important part of your core training routine because they strengthen the posterior chain. The posterior chain is made up of muscles in the back side of your body, including the gluteus, hamstrings, and lower back. These muscles are important in daily life activities, such as jumping, running, sitting down, and standing up.

A strong posterior chain has many benefits, including enhancing overall athleticism, strength, and explosiveness, as well as improving the appearance of the back side of the body and lifting the butt.

TABLE

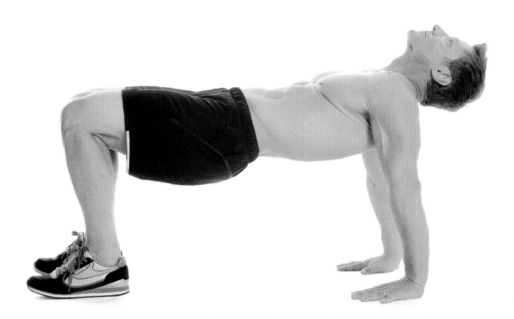

> **SKILL LEVEL: Beginner**

> **MODIFICATION: None**

The most basic reverse plank is the reverse table with a static hold.

KEY PERFORMANCE POINTS

- Sit down on the floor with your knees bent and your hands placed directly underneath your shoulders with your fingertips facing your butt.
- Press into your palms and feet, and lift your hips up so that your body creates a straight line from your knee to your shoulder in a table position.
- Let your head fall back slightly, and look straight up.

COMMON FAULTS

- Sagging hips
- Bent elbows
- Wrists not in line with shoulders

PAYOFF This plank tones the gluteus and hamstrings while stretching the chest and shoulders.

REVERSE PLANK

REVERSE PLANK

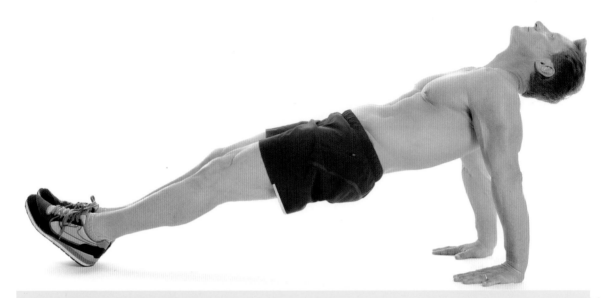

> **SKILL LEVEL: Advanced**

> **MODIFICATION: None**

The full version of reverse plank requires a strong core and activation of the gluteus and hamstrings as you maintain a static hold.

KEY PERFORMANCE POINTS

- Sit down on the floor with your legs straight out in front of you and your hands placed directly underneath your shoulders with your fingertips facing your butt.

- Press into your palms and feet, and lift your hips up so that your body creates a straight line from your shoulders to your feet. Push into your big toes, and keep your inner thighs active and engaged to help maintain the hold.

- Let your head fall back slightly, and look straight up.

COMMON FAULTS

- Sagging hips
- Bent elbows
- Wrists not in line with shoulders

PAYOFF This plank strengthens the gluteus, hamstrings, lower back, wrists, and inner thighs while stretching the chest and shoulders.

LEG LIFT

REVERSE PLANK

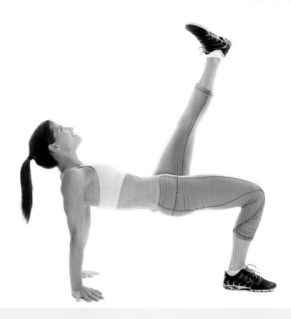

> **SKILL LEVEL: Intermediate**

> **MODIFICATION: Perform in full reverse plank (to make it harder)**

Here one point of support is removed in the reverse table leg lift for an extra core and gluteus challenge. Maintain a static hold on each side.

KEY PERFORMANCE POINTS

- Sit down on the floor with your knees bent and your hands placed directly underneath your shoulders with your fingertips facing your butt.

- Press into your palms and feet. Lift your hips up, and then lift one leg straight up as you press through your heel and squeeze your quadriceps.

- Let your head fall back slightly and look straight up at the lifted foot.

COMMON FAULTS

- Sagging hips

- Bent elbows

- Bent extended knee

- Wrists not in line with shoulders

- One hip dropped out of alignment

PAYOFF This plank isolates the gluteus for maximum toning.

TABLE KICKS

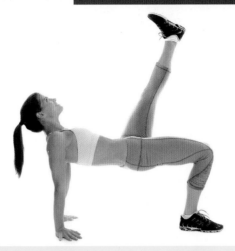

> **SKILL LEVEL: Intermediate**

> **MODIFICATION: Perform in full reverse plank (to make it harder), or target the obliques and kick the leg across the body toward the opposite knee (to make it harder)**

Take the reverse table leg lift one step further by adding more movement. In this variation, you will alternate reps of kicking one foot away and then the other.

KEY PERFORMANCE POINTS

- Sit down on the floor with your knees bent and hands placed directly underneath your shoulders with your fingertips facing your butt.

- Press into your palms and feet, and lift your hips up. Then, kick one leg straight up. Lower it to the starting position, and repeat on the other side.

- Let your head fall back slightly, and look straight up at the lifted foot.

COMMON FAULTS

- Sagging hips
- Bent elbows
- Bent extended knee
- Wrists not in line with shoulders
- One hip dropped out of alignment

PAYOFF The movement in this plank creates an extra core challenge and elevates the heart rate.

TABLE CRUNCH TWIST

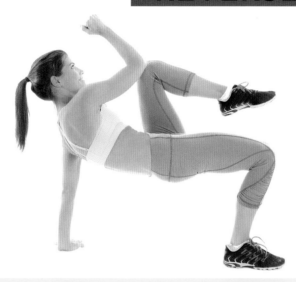

> **SKILL LEVEL: Intermediate**

> **MODIFICATION: None**

This table variation adds a knee lift and a twisting crunch. Repeat reps on both sides.

KEY PERFORMANCE POINTS

- Sit down on the floor with your knees bent and your hands placed directly underneath your shoulders with your fingertips facing your butt.

- Press into your palms and feet, and lift your hips up into table position. Draw one knee into your chest, and lift the opposite elbow.

- Move through the reps of a twisted crunch by drawing your knee and elbow together and then extending your foot away.

COMMON FAULTS

- Sagging hips
- Bent elbow on the supported hand
- Wrists not in line with shoulders
- One hip dropped out of alignment

PAYOFF This plank tones the butt and works the abs.

BRIDGE

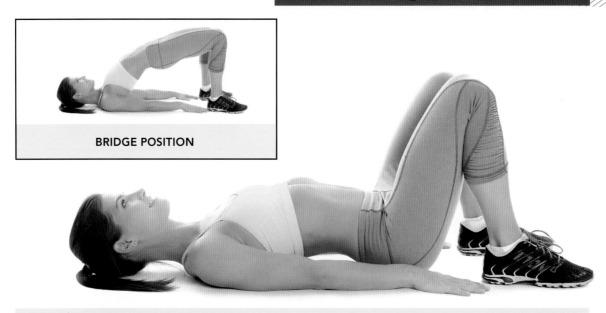

BRIDGE POSITION

> **SKILL LEVEL: Beginner**

> **MODIFICATION: Add in hip dips by lowering the hips to the floor and lifting back up again (to make it harder)**

Bridge is a gentle backbend that stretches the chest and the shoulders while it strengthens the back side of the body. Maintain a static hold in bridge.

KEY PERFORMANCE POINTS

- Lie back on the floor, and bend your knees, placing your feet on the floor as close to your butt as possible and hip width apart.

- Press into your feet and arms to lift up through your hips until your thighs are nearly parallel with the floor. Engaging through your gluteus compresses your lower back, so press into your heels and use strong thighs to maintain the hold.

- Walk your shoulder blades together to take the pressure off of your neck and spine as you lift the chin away from your chest and press into the back of your head.

COMMON FAULTS

- Flat chest and sagging hips
- Knees out too wide
- Overly engaged gluteus

PAYOFF This plank promotes a healthy spine.

FOREARM

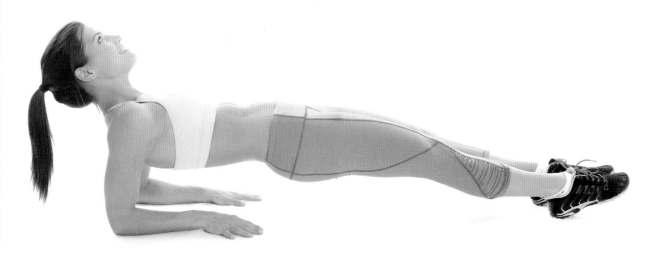

> **SKILL LEVEL: Advanced**

> **MODIFICATION: Bend the knees (to make it easier)**

This is the most difficult variation of reverse plank. Here, you will take the reverse plank down to the forearms while maintaining a static hold.

KEY PERFORMANCE POINTS

- Sit down on the floor with your legs straight out in front of you. Prop yourself up on your forearms with your elbows directly under your shoulders.
- Press into your forearms, and lift your hips up so that your body creates a straight line from your shoulders to feet. Push into your big toes, and keep your inner thighs active and engaged to help maintain the hold.
- Let your head fall back slightly, and look straight up.

COMMON FAULTS

- Sagging hips
- Bent knees
- Elbows not in line with shoulders

PAYOFF Feel the fire in your shoulders and hamstrings with this plank.

SLIDE-THROUGH

REVERSE PLANK

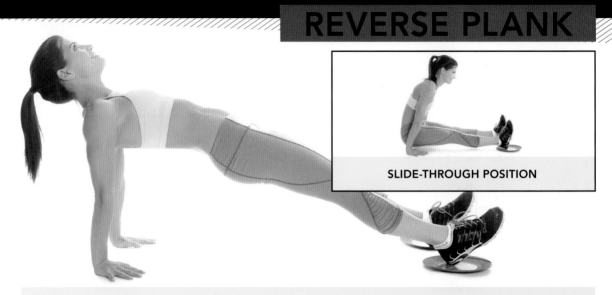

SLIDE-THROUGH POSITION

> **SKILL LEVEL: Advanced**

> **MODIFICATION: Perform the movement from a table position without the gliding disks by pulling the hips through and straightening the legs (to make it easier)**

Adding the gliding disks to reverse planks allows you to move through reps of a reverse sit-up movement and is a great combination of front and back side body toning.

KEY PERFORMANCE POINTS

- Sit down on the floor with your legs straight out in front of you. Put your heels in the center of two gliding disks and your hands directly underneath your shoulders with your fingertips facing your butt.

- Press into your palms and feet, and lift your hips up so that your body creates a straight line from your shoulders to feet.

- Dip your hips down and pull your butt back between your hands. Then, press into your palms, lift your hips, and squeeze through your quads to return to the starting position.

COMMON FAULTS

- Sagging hips

- Bent elbows

- Wrists not in line with shoulders

PAYOFF This one exercise strengthens the front and back side of the core.

CHAPTER TWELVE

STRETCHING PLANKS

GENTLY STRETCH, STRENGTHEN, AND LENGTHEN

The planks in this chapter are designed to stretch your body while still gently working the core. They are a great addition to the warmup and cooldown portions of your workout. These planks will increase your flexibility while helping to stretch and lengthen muscles, assisting in recovery from workouts.

MERMAID

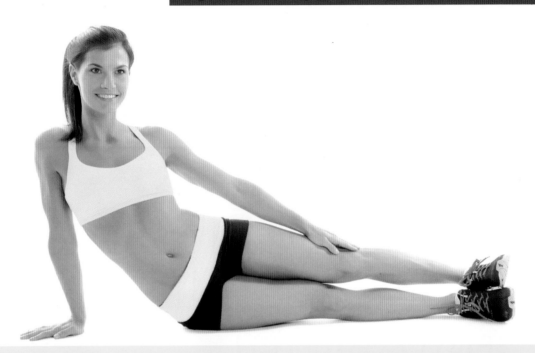

> **SKILL LEVEL: Beginner**

> **MODIFICATION: Bend the knees and bring the feet back behind you (to make it easier)**

Mermaid is a wonderful stretch for the side body. Maintain a static hold in this position.

KEY PERFORMANCE POINTS

- Lie down on your side, and prop yourself up on one forearm.
- Press the opposite palm into the floor in front of you to give you the leverage to lift up from your forearm to your palm.
- Press your grounded palm into the floor, and relax your shoulder away from your ear.

COMMON FAULTS

- Bent elbow
- Improper alignment of shoulders and wrists
- Hips rotated forwards or backward

PAYOFF This plank lengthens and stretches the side body.

REVOLVED SIDE
STRETCHING PLANK

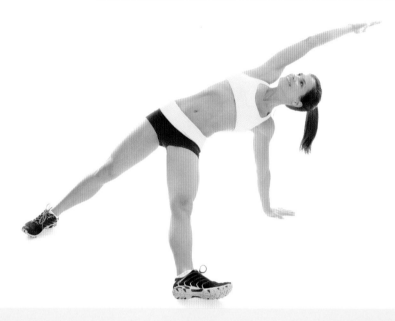

> **SKILL LEVEL: Beginner**

> **MODIFICATION: Bring the threaded foot closer to the grounded foot (to make it easier) or bring the threaded foot closer to the shoulder (to make it harder)**

Revolved side plank provides a stretch for the hips, hip flexors, shoulders, and chest. Maintain a static hold on each side.

KEY PERFORMANCE POINTS

- Get into a full plank position with your body in a straight line with your shoulders stacked over your wrists.

- Thread your right foot under your body and over to your left.

- Transfer your body weight onto your right hand. Lift your left hand up and over your head, pressing into your right hand and right leg to keep your hips lifted. Open your chest.

COMMON FAULTS

- Sagging hips
- Bent elbow
- Improper alignment of shoulders and wrists

PAYOFF This plank opens the hips, shoulders, and chest.

MODIFIED SIDE WITH A REACH

STRETCHING PLANK

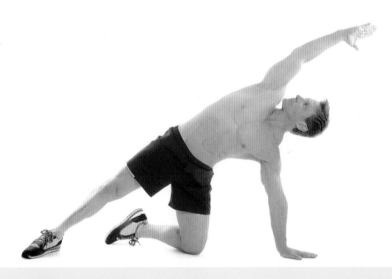

> **SKILL LEVEL: Beginner**

> **MODIFICATION: None**

This grounded variation of side plank is a great way to open and stretch the side body as well as the abdominal wall and the chest. Maintain a static hold on each side.

KEY PERFORMANCE POINTS

- Get into a side plank with your bottom knee grounded on the floor and your top leg extended out. Bring the shin of the grounded knee back behind you for more stabilization.

- Stack your shoulder over the grounded hand, and then reach the top arm up and overhead. Try to rotate your chest and gaze upward.

- Reach through the tips of the extended fingers, and press down into the blade of the extended leg.

COMMON FAULTS

- Shoulders rolled forward
- Improper alignment of shoulders and wrists

PAYOFF This plank stretches the abdominal wall, chest, and side body.

140 // ULTIMATE PLANK FITNESS

MODIFIED SIDE

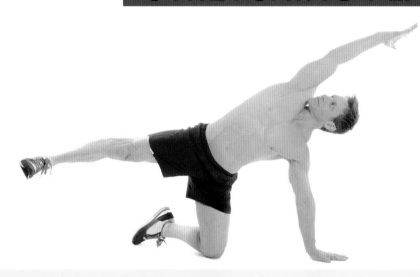

> **SKILL LEVEL: Intermediate**

> **MODIFICATION: None**

Modified side plank becomes an exercise in balance and stability when a leg lift is added. This will challenge the obliques and build strength in the hips while still providing a stretch. Maintain a static hold on both sides.

KEY PERFORMANCE POINTS

- Get into a side plank with your bottom knee grounded on the floor and your top leg extended out. You can kickstand your bottom leg for more support.
- Stack the shoulder over the grounded hand, and then reach your top arm up and overhead. Try to rotate your chest and gaze upward.
- Reach through the tips of the extended fingers, and lift the extended leg up so that there is a straight line from your hip to your heel.

COMMON FAULTS

- Shoulder rolled forward
- Improper alignment of shoulders and wrists
- Lifted leg not parallel with hip

PAYOFF This plank builds strength in the outer hip while also developing balance and stability.

BOUND MODIFIED
STRETCHING PLANK

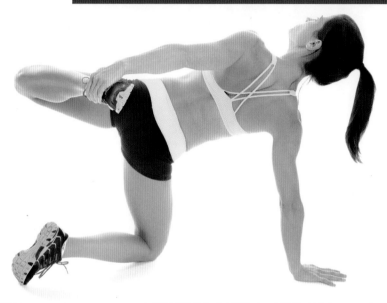

> **SKILL LEVEL: Intermediate**

> **MODIFICATION: None**

This variation of modified side plank has multiple benefits. It's a backbend that opens up the upper back, chest, and shoulders. The bend also provides a stretch for the hip flexors and quadriceps. Maintain a static hold on both sides.

KEY PERFORMANCE POINTS

- Get into a side plank with your bottom knee grounded on the floor and your top leg extended out. You can kickstand your bottom leg for more support.

- Float the extended leg up, and bend your knee. Reach the extended arm back to the top of your foot. Kick your hand against your foot, and gently press your hips forward.

- Stack your shoulder over the grounded hand, and press into the floor to stabilize. Try to rotate your chest and gaze upward.

COMMON FAULTS

- Improper alignment of shoulders and wrists

PAYOFF This plank stretches the hip flexors and quads, and provides a gentle backbend.

SIDE-TO-SIDE GATE
STRETCHING PLANK

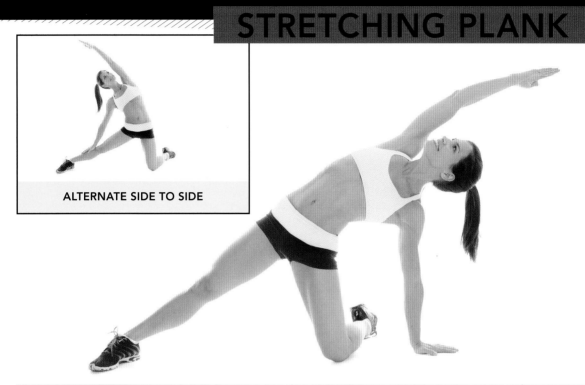

ALTERNATE SIDE TO SIDE

> **SKILL LEVEL: Beginner**
> **MODIFICATION: Use a block under the hands (to make it easier)**

This stretching plank involves movement as you flow side to side to strengthen and stretch the obliques. Repeat reps of this on both sides.

KEY PERFORMANCE POINTS

- Get into a kneeling position on the floor, and extend your right leg out. Press into the outside edge of your foot.
- Reach your left hand down to your left shin and your right hand overhead. Keep your left hip stacked over your left knee.
- Engage through your obliques, and change directions. Float your left hand down to the floor, and reach your right hand overhead. Try to open your chest and slightly lift your gaze as you reach overhead.

COMMON FAULTS

- Hip out of alignment with grounded knee

PAYOFF This plank builds strength in the obliques while it stretches the side body.

FLOWING

> **SKILL LEVEL: Beginner**

> **MODIFICATION: None**

This plank variation moves you through a flowing motion of going from plank to downward-facing dog to upward-facing dog to stretching the back side and front side of the body.

KEY PERFORMANCE POINTS

- Get into a full plank position with your hands under your shoulders and a straight line from your head to your heels.

- Press into your palms, and lift your hips to come into what's called downward-facing dog. In your "down dog," squeeze your quads to sink your heels down to the floor, keeping your arms long and straight as you relax your shoulders away from your ears. Gaze between your knees to keep your neck long.

- Come back out to full plank, and drop your hips down to come into what's called upward-facing dog. Untuck your toes, and press into the tops of your feet as you gently pull your hips and chest through. Roll your shoulders down and back.

COMMON FAULTS

- Bent elbows and knees in "down dog"

- Bent elbows in "up dog"

- Tucked toes in "up dog," which compresses the lower back

- Rounding of your shoulders in "up dog"

PAYOFF This is a total body stretch. This plank hits the hamstrings, calves, achilles tendons, abdomen, chest, and more.

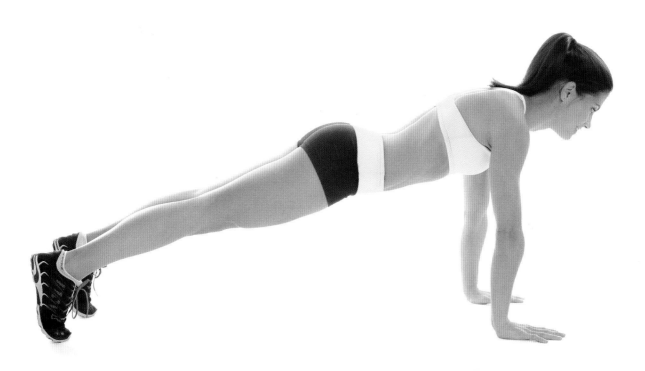

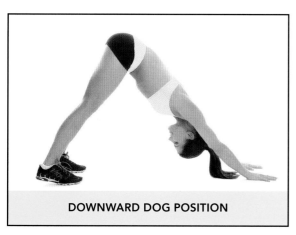

DOWNWARD DOG POSITION

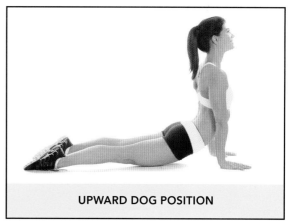

UPWARD DOG POSITION

CHAPTER THIRTEEN

EXTRA-CREDIT
PLANKS

COMBINE EQUIPMENT AND SURFACES FOR THE ULTIMATE CHALLENGE

Try these three planks for extra credit. These tough planks combine multiple unstable surfaces for the ultimate core challenge. Build your strength, and work your way up to these planks.

MEDICINE BALL AND BOSU

FULL PLANK

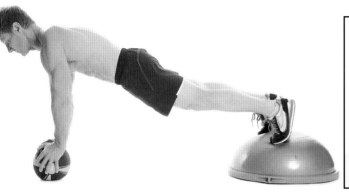

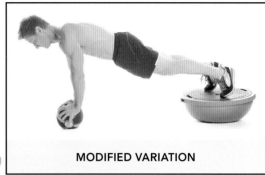

MODIFIED VARIATION

> **SKILL LEVEL:** Advanced

> **MODIFICATION:** Lift one leg (to make it harder) or flip the BOSU to the ball side and place the feet on the flat side (to make it harder)

In this balancing full plank, the hands are on a medicine ball, and the feet are on the BOSU Trainer as you maintain a static hold.

KEY PERFORMANCE POINTS

- Stack your shoulders directly over your wrists. Place your hands on either side of the medicine ball, and press into your palms.

- Place your toes in the center of the BOSU Trainer, and get into a straight body position from your head to your heels with feet hip width apart.

- Maintain a tight core while squeezing through your quads and chest to support the core and make the hold easier.

COMMON FAULTS

- Sagging lower back
- Butt lifted higher than your heels and head
- Bent knees
- Improper alignment of shoulders and wrists

PAYOFF This plank develops shoulder stabilization and total body control.

STABILITY BALL

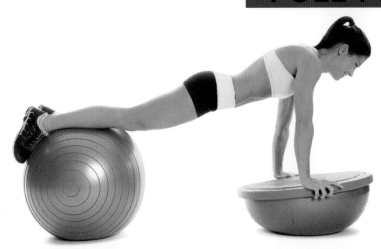

> **SKILL LEVEL: Advanced**

> **MODIFICATION: Flip the BOSU so that the flat side is on the floor (to make it easier)**

In this balancing full plank, the hands are on a BOSU Trainer as the feet balance on a stability ball.

KEY PERFORMANCE POINTS

- Stack your shoulders directly over your wrists. Place your hands on either side of the BOSU Trainer, and grip the handles.

- Working one leg at a time, place your shins and tops of your feet on the top of a stability ball. The closer you place the ball to your knees and thighs, the more support you'll have.

- Maintain a tight core while squeezing through the quads and chest to support the core and make the hold easier.

COMMON FAULTS

- Sagging lower back

- Butt lifted higher than the head and heels

- Improper alignment of shoulders and wrists

PAYOFF This plank is the ultimate in building core control.

BOSU + GLIDING DISK MOUNTAIN CLIMBER

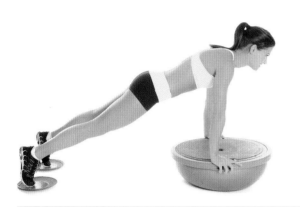
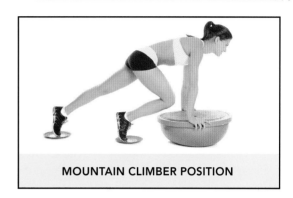

MOUNTAIN CLIMBER POSITION

> **SKILL LEVEL: Advanced**

> **MODIFICATION: Flip the BOSU so that the flat side is on the floor (to make it easier)**

In this full plank, the hands are on a BOSU Trainer as you "mountain climb" the feet on gliding disks.

KEY PERFORMANCE POINTS

- Stack your shoulders directly over your wrists. Place your hands on either side of the BOSU Trainer, and grip the handles.
- Place the balls of your feet on gliding disks with your heels lifted and pressed back.
- Draw one knee into your chest, and then press it back into full plank. Alternate sides. This is called the mountain climber.
- This is a quick movement; you should feel like you are jogging your knees into your chest.

COMMON FAULTS

- Shortening of the plank stance
- Bent elbows
- Improper alignment of shoulders and wrists

PAYOFF This combination of movements gives you both cardio and core.

SAMPLE WORKOUTS

Ready to put these planks into practice and build the strongest core of your life as you change the shape of your body? Get ready to feel the burn with these ten workouts that link together a series of planks from the chapters in this book. The workouts range from beginner to advanced and are all around five minutes in duration.

WORKOUT 1: BEGINNER

The focus of this workout is to build up the amount of time you are able to stay in a full plank. As the 15-second holds get easier, start to increase the amount of time you are in the plank over the course of 1 minute. For example, start at 15-seconds in the full plank hold, with five seconds rest and repeated three times, and then increase to 25-seconds in the full plank, with 5-seconds rest and repeated once. Continue to increase the plank hold time until you are able to hold a plank for a full minute.

Each variation should total 1 minute

VARIATION ONE: 15-second full plank (page 15), 5-second rest. *Repeat two times.*

VARIATION TWO: 15-second right side plank (page 36), 5-second rest. *Repeat two times.*

VARIATION TWO: 15-second left side plank (page 36), 5-seconds rest. *Repeat two times.*

VARIATION FOUR: 15-second forearm plank (page 49), 5-seconds rest. *Repeat two times.*

VARIATION FIVE: 15-second bridge (page 134), 5-seconds rest. *Repeat two times.*

WORKOUT 2: INTERMEDIATE

These variations are rep-based and add movement to the plank.

VARIATION ONE:

10 knee to chest planks (page 16) *five on each leg*

10 twisted knee to chest planks (page 17)

10 mountain climber planks (page 18)

Repeat this set three times.

VARIATION TWO:

10 side plank with foot taps (page 39) *ten on each leg*

5 side plank hip dips (page 38) *five on each side*

10 side forearm stability ball planks (page 70) *ten on each side*

Repeat this set three times.

VARIATION THREE:

10 forearm plank knee taps (page 51)

10 forearm plank hip drops (page 52) *five on each side*

10 plank walks (page 26) *high plank to forearm plank*

Repeat this set three times.

WORKOUT 3: ADVANCED

This advanced bodyweight workout features movement and single arm/leg balancing.

8 pulsing full planks (page 24) *eight on each leg*

8 side planks with knee crunches (page 44) *eight on each leg*

8 table crunch twists (page 133) *eight on each leg*

8 push-up side planks (page 46) *four on each side*

30-second rocking forearm plank (page 50)

8 dolphin plank push-ups (page 56)

Repeat this set three times.

WORKOUT 4: STABILITY BALL

This workout requires your stability ball; get ready for a circuit-based workout that will challenge the core.

30-second stability ball forearm plank (page 69)

15-second stability ball balancing plank (page 71)

10 stability ball knee tucks (page 72)

15-second stability ball side forearm plank (page 70) *15-seconds on each side*

30-second stability ball reverse plank (page 78)

Repeat this set three times.

WORKOUT 5: BOSU TRAINER

You'll work with both sides of the BOSU Trainer in this rep-themed workout that will have you moving and twisting.

10 BOSU plank walks (page 83)

15-second BOSU side forearm plank (page 84)
15-seconds on each side

10 knee to chests from flipped BOSU full plank (page 16, but on the BOSU) *five on each leg*

10 twisted knee to chests from flipped BOSU full plank (page 17, but on the BOSU)
five on each leg

Repeat this set three times.

WORKOUT 6: MEDICINE BALL

This medicine ball workout features a combination of static and moving planks.

8 pulsing leg lift medicine ball planks (page 90)
eight on each leg

30-second medicine ball plank hold (page 87)

8 medicine ball cheetah crunches (page 91)
four on each leg

8 rolling medicine ball planks (page 89) *four on each side*

Repeat this set three times.

WORKOUT 7: WEIGHTS

Perform this set of short planks with weights to strengthen the core while also toning the entire body.

12 dumbbell plank rows (page 98)
twelve on each arm

12 dumbbell tricep kickbacks (page 100)
twelve on each arm

15-second weighted side plank (page 103)
15-seconds on each side

12 stability ball chest presses (page 105)

12 stability ball overhead extensions (page 107)

Repeat this set two times.

WORKOUT 8: GLIDING DISK

All you need is a set of gliding disks to get your heart rate up and your core burning. This is a tough one.

15 forearm plank gliding body saws (page 118)

10 knees to chest planks (page 120)
ten on each leg

10 gliding disk crunches or V-ups (page 123 or 124)

10 twisted knee to chests (page 121)
ten on each leg

Repeat this set three times.

WORKOUT 9: MIXED STATIC

This workout features static holds while utilizing a mixture of equipment and plank variations.

10-second one arm plank (page 25)
10-seconds on each arm

20-second full side plank (page 36)
20-seconds each side, option to add a leg lift or tree variation

30-second forearm plank (page 49)

20-second side forearm plank (page 59)
20-seconds on each arm, with an option to add a leg lift

10-second spinal balancing plank (page 20)
10-seconds on each arm

30-second modified side plank with a reach
(page 140) *30-seconds on each side*

WORKOUT 10: MIXED MOVEMENT

This workout features movement-based plank exercises while utilizing a mixture of equipment.

10 three point knee to chests (page 27)
five on each leg

10 table kicks (page 132)
five on each leg

10 plank jacks (page 112)

5 BOSU side forearm with knee crunches
(page 85) *five each side*

10 BOSU gliding disk twisted knee to chest
planks (page 121) *ten each side*

Repeat this set three times.

INDEX

ACKNOWLEDGMENTS

First and foremost, to my editor Jill Alexander. Thank you for bringing this project to the table and for believing in me. I couldn't have done this without your guidance every step of the way.

David Martinell, your creative vision truly made this book come alive in print. Thank you for making the book even more beautiful and dynamic than I could have hoped.

Renae Haines, thank you for all of the behind the scenes and logistical work. You are a super star.

To my photographer Wanda Koch, it is a joy to know you and you bring so much light to every person and every project you touch. Thank you for your time, your energy, and your belief in our work.

Mom and Dad, you fostered independence and drive in me from a young age. Mom, thank you for giving me my love for language and words (and grammar!). Dad, thank you for always knowing just the right time to say, "I'm proud of you." The support you two have shown me throughout my life has truly been unconditional.

Mema, you opened me up to a world of both abundant love and possibility. I cherish every moment we have shared and every memory we've made.

Brandon, your steadfast friendship and encouragement has meant more to me than I will ever be able to express.

Dorie, for being there every step of the way during a year of unprecedented growth and change, thank you. Your friendship is a treasure.

Mandy, your guidance has been unbelievably helpful over the last few years as I have grown personally and professionally. I am forever grateful for you for keeping me clear on my path.

Marc, you were the perfect partner for photography for the book. Thank you for your time and enthusiasm for the project.

And to my Sullie girl, your sweet soul brings me so much happiness and so many smiles.

ABOUT THE AUTHOR

Jennifer DeCurtins is the creator of the popular healthy lifestyle blog Peanut Butter Runner, where she shares daily updates about food, fitness, and yoga. An experienced fitness professional, Jennifer is a NASM certified personal trainer, 200-hour registered yoga teacher, CrossFit coach, and group exercise instructor. She also writes a running and fitness website for the Charlotte Observer. Jennifer lives in Charlotte, North Carolina, with her golden retriever Sullie.